Transmasculinity on Television

This book explores how television and streaming services portray transgender characters who identify as male or nonbinary in television media.

Transmasculinity on Television takes a closer look at transmasculine and nonbinary characters on broadcast, cable, and streaming services between 2000 and 2021. Significant changes have occurred since the release of the 1999 film *Boys Don't Cry*, and in particular through the increase in transgender producers, writers, and actors playing those roles. While a great deal of research has been published on gay, lesbian, and female transgender characters, very little analysis has been done on trans male representation in American media. This book examines the history of how film and television have portrayed transgender characters, how these depictions have developed over time, and what impact these representations may have on audience attitudes.

This accessible and engaging study is suitable for students and scholars in gender studies, media studies, and LGBTQ studies.

Patrice A. Oppliger (she/her/hers) received her doctorate in mass communication from the University of Alabama. She is currently an assistant professor of media science at Boston University. Her research focuses on media effects (particularly adolescent viewers), humor, and gender studies.

Focus on Global Gender and Sexuality

Pornography, Indigeneity and Neocolonialism
Tim Gregory

Reading Iraqi Women's Novels in English Translation
Iraqi Women's Stories
Ruth Abou Rached

Gender Hierarchy of Masculinity and Femininity during the Chinese Cultural Revolution
Revolutionary Opera Films
Zhuying Li

Representations of Lethal Gender-Based Violence in Italy Between Journalism and Literature
Femminicidio Narratives
Nicoletta Mandolini

LGBTQI Digital Media Activism and Counter-Hate Speech in Italy
Sara Gabai

Transmasculinity on Television
Patrice A. Oppliger

What Do We Know About the Effects of Pornography After Fifty Years of Academic Research?
Alan McKee, Katerina Litsou, Paul Byron and Roger Ingham

For more information about this series, please visit: www.routledge.com/Focus-on-Global-Gender-and-Sexuality/book-series/FGGS

Transmasculinity on Television

Patrice A. Oppliger

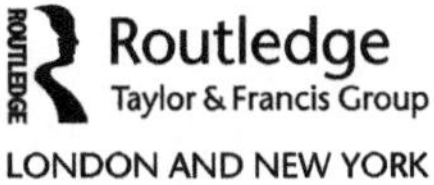
LONDON AND NEW YORK

First published 2022
by Routledge
4 Park Square, Milton Park, Abingdon, Oxon OX14 4RN

and by Routledge
605 Third Avenue, New York, NY 10158

Routledge is an imprint of the Taylor & Francis Group, an informa business

British Library Cataloguing-in-Publication Data
A catalogue record for this book is available from the British Library

Library of Congress Cataloging-in-Publication Data
A catalog record has been requested for this book

ISBN: 978-1-032-06898-5 (hbk)
ISBN: 978-1-032-06899-2 (pbk)
ISBN: 978-1-003-20440-4 (ebk)

DOI: 10.4324/9781003204404

Typeset in Times new Roman
by Apex CoVantage, LLC

Contents

	Preface	vi
1	Introduction	1
2	The Importance of Standpoint	12
3	Transgender Across Genres	23
4	How to Be Television Trans	46
5	Allies and Adversaries	71
	Afterword	91
	Appendix: Character Chart	96
	References	98
	Index	110

Preface

Ellis (2020) defined "transgender" to mean "people whose gender identity and/or gender expression differs from what is typically associated with the sex they were assigned at birth." According to a Gallup poll, 0.6% of American adults identify as transgender (Jones, 2021). Steinmetz (2014) argued that a small representative of the population can make it harder for groups like transgender individuals to gain acceptance. The 0.6% might not seem significant, but it represents as many as 1.5 million Americans, not including those under 18 who identify as transgender.

Identifying as transgender in the United States comes with great risks, such as discrimination and threats of physical, mental, and emotional harm. Data show transgender individuals face higher rates of unemployment, harassment, suicide, incarceration, murder, and homelessness than other Americans (Grant, Mottet, & Tanis, 2011). While Donaghue (2020) reported a recent "horrific spike" in violence against transgender individuals, these statistics are likely even higher because law enforcement and the news media often underreport victims by misgendering them (e.g., using their deadnames to classify their gender identity). For transgender youth, statistics are especially grim. More than 60% of transgender and nonbinary youth reported self-harming in the past 12 months, while 75% reported symptoms of anxiety disorder (Paley, 2020). A study by the American Academy of Pediatrics noted alarming rates of suicide attempts among transgender youth, with the highest rates for transgender boys (Hassanein, 2018). According to Rapaport (2019), when schools required students to use facilities based on their sex assigned at birth, sexual assault of transgender girls forced to use boys' restrooms increased 26%. Moreover, some transgender youth reported avoiding using restrooms, which resulted in insufficient fluid intake, urinary tract infections, and impacted bowels, as well as overall school avoidance.

Although this book is not political in nature, a review of partisan issues gives insight into individuals' perceptions of gender. Just over half (56%)

of US adults and nearly all (90%) of conservative Republicans believe that sex assigned at birth determines whether someone is a man or a woman, according a Pew Research Center poll (cited in Minkin & Brown, 2021). In contrast, younger, more educated, more democratic-leaning individuals believe gender can vary. Further, 60% of Democrats report that society has not gone far enough in accepting transgender people; however, 57% of Republicans continue to believe that society has "gone too far." The Trump administration acted on and perpetuated this belief, banning transgender people from enlisting and serving in the US military and attempting to remove health care protections for transgender individuals (Schmidt, 2020). Sparked by North Carolina's HB2 "bathroom bill" in 2016, a Pew Research study reported that a record number of state-level bills in 2021 have "sought to limit definitions of gender to the sex people are assigned at birth" (Minkin & Brown, 2021). At least 28 state legislatures are taking up anti-transgender bills to bar transgender youth from participating in sports and access to medical treatment (Hansen, 2021).

Importance of Media Portrayals

Research demonstrates that contact with individuals who openly identify as LGBTQ in their private, public, and/or professional lives can influence societal attitudes. In other words, knowing someone who is transgender is correlated with the acceptance that a person's gender can differ from their sex at birth (Minkin & Brown, 2021). While the number of people who report knowing a transgender person is steadily increasing (42% in 2021, up from 8% in 2013), it is still a minority (Minkin & Brown, 2021). Individuals who report not knowing a transgender person likely learned about transgender issues from the media. In fact, for both cisgender (i.e., identifying with the gender they were assigned at birth) and transgender people, the media is likely the main source of information about transgender issues (McInroy & Craig, 2015). Along with encouraging contact with people who openly self-identify as transgender, Blair (2019) advocated for increasing accurate media representations to effectively reduce transgender prejudice. This is especially important since Halberstam (2018) noted that transness is still seen as an aberration, and at times characters can appear "mad, bad, and dangerous" (p. 92).

When I discussed writing this book with friends and even fellow academics, nearly everyone asks, "Are there any transgender men on TV?" There have been significantly fewer portrayals and less scholarship published on individuals who were assigned female at birth and who now identify as male or nonbinary. In this analysis, I use heinz's (2016) definition of "transmasculine" to mean "self-identification toward maleness, manhood, or masculine or identifying on a male spectrum or masculine gender expression, and do not simply mimic cis male characteristics." The absence of research on the topic, particularly the lack of emphasis on transmasculine characters, in addition to the importance of media representation, is my motivation for writing this book. My analysis is focused on mainstream television produced for a mainstream audience who likely lacks direct knowledge of transmasculinity in real life.

Final Thoughts

Before I begin my analyses, I would like to address sensitivity issues related to my cisgender status. I acknowledge that as a cis woman, I cannot know what it is to be transgender or what effect transgender portrayals can have on transgender audiences. I can only see the topic through the lens of my years researching media content and media effects. My interest in media effects stems from having grown up on a farm in rural Nebraska. With the lack of diversity in my community, television was my window into a broader awareness beyond the exclusively white and (apparently) cis, straight world I saw around me.

Halberstam (2018) noted that historically there has been variability in terminology describing gender-diverse individuals. According to Serano (2007), "Most non-trans people are unfamiliar with the words that we in the transgender community use to describe ourselves, our experiences, and our most pressing issues" (p. 29). I reached out to transgender scholars and therapists to help with my understanding of the subject and to assist me in including the most sensitive, accurate, and up-to-date terminology. A huge thanks to Dax Ebaden, Brett Herb, and Jake Reeves for their help on this project. I also want to thank my graduate assistants from Boston University—Mel Medeiros, Shelby Muschler, and Morgan Anderson—for their hard work.

1 Introduction

According to Abrams (2020), gender essentialism assumes that qualities attributed to women and men are linked to chromosomes and other biological traits. Seeing these qualities as fixed, intrinsic, and innate denies an individual's ability to self-determine gender identity and gender presentation. Scholars have traced this notion back to Plato's philosophy of essentialism (Abrams, 2020). By the mid-20th century, according to Abrams (2020), it was scientifically proven "that sex doesn't necessarily determine or indicate anything conclusive or permanent about an individual's gender identity, personality, or preferences." Findings such as these have not deterred religious and conservative political groups. In fact, discrimination and bigotry have increased as transgender issues have gained more media coverage. Gallagher and Bodenhausen (2021) argued that the increased visibility of transgender individuals challenges a "dominant cultural model of gender," the result of which leads to the perpetuation of sex binaries that remain unchangeable from birth to adulthood.

Just as scientific and medical studies have advanced our understanding of sex and gender, language describing gender identity has also evolved. "Transsexual," one of the earliest terms to describe gender variance, was added to the American lexicon in 1949 (Whittle, 2010). Critics have since found the word "transsexual" to be offensive and stigmatizing because it incorrectly labels transgender people in a way that makes them seem mentally ill or sexually deviant (Abrams, 2019). The term "transgender" (coined in 1971) is currently seen as more inclusive and affirming because it embraces individuals' experience whether or not they pursue medical changes to affirm their gender. Transgender is often used as "an umbrella term for gender-variant bodies," according to Halberstam (2018). "Cisgender," in contrast, refers to someone whose current gender identity is the same as the one they were assigned at birth (Blair, 2019). These terms have long and sordid histories that reflect "multiple, sometimes overlapping, sometimes even contested meanings" (Stryker & Currah, 2014, p. 1).

DOI: 10.4324/9781003204404-1

Examples of transgender and nonbinary gender identification have been around for millennia, tracing back to the Gala priests of Sumer around 2450 BC, who identified as neither male nor female (Roscoe, 1996). In the modern era, Christine Jorgensen signified the first public figure in the United States to undergo gender reassignment surgery in 1952. In 1976, Renee Richards's surgical transitioning made headlines. Richards challenged the United States Tennis Association's genetic screening requirement for women's tennis players. Although she lost in the first round, she was allowed to play in the women's US Open tournament. In the popular culture realm, Laverne Cox, famous for her role as a transfeminine character Sophia on Netflix's *Orange Is the New Black* (2013–2019), became the first openly transgender person to appear on the covers of *Time* (Westcott, 2014) and *Cosmo* (Wong, 2018) magazines. Caitlyn Jenner's transition announcement in 2015 prompted even more media coverage. That year, hers was the second most Googled name (Sebastian, 2015), her interview on ABC's *20/20* attracted over 20 million viewers (Berman, 2015), and she broke the *Guinness Book of World Records* for amassing one million Twitter followers in the shortest amount of time (Parkinson, 2015).

Transmasculine individuals, on the other hand, have received far less attention. One of the earliest public transmasculine figures was Billy Tipton, a jazz musician and band leader from the 1930s–1970s. Although he was assigned female at birth (AFAB), he lived as a man, socially transitioning without surgery or hormones (Green, 2016). His gender status was not revealed to most people he knew, including many of his wives and three adopted sons, until his death in 1989. According to Alex Schmider (2021), the associate director of GLAAD's Transgender Representation, "The subsequent media attention was almost uniformly dehumanizing and disrespectful, with media stories and books misgendering Billy and accusing him of deceiving his family and the public." In 2011, Chaz Bono's appearance on *Dancing with the Stars* marked the first openly transgender man to star on a major network television show for something "unrelated to being transgender" (Advocate, 2011b). Most recently, in 2021, Elliot Page became the first openly transgender man to appear on the cover of *Time* magazine.

Transgender Cinema Studies

Judith Butler's (1990) frequently cited book *Gender Trouble: Feminism and the Subversion of Identity* was influential in developing the interdisciplinary field of transgender studies and gender performativity. According to Stryker and Currah (2014), editors of the first issue of *TSQ: Transgender Studies Quarterly*, this theoretical framework provides "a broadly inclusive rubric for describing expressions of gender that vary from expected norms" (p. 5).

In order to study media representations, scholars have employed transgender cinema studies with the understanding that gender identity is socially constructed rather than a stable, fixed phenomenon. Henry (2019) noted that in the past two decades, transgender studies has emerged as a discipline led by pioneers such as Susan Stryker and Jack Halberstam. A "new generation of screen and media scholars" includes Helen Hok-Sze Leung, Cáel M. Keegan, Eliza Steinbock, and Akkadia Ford.

Halberstam (2005) identified three categories that describe various queer representations in cinema: trivialization (queer life is "dismissed as non-representative and inconsequential"), stabilization (queer narratives are "defused by establishing the queer narrative as strange, uncharacteristic, even pathological"), and rationalization ("filmmaker finds reasonable explanations for behavior that may seem dangerous and outrageous"). Typical Hollywood portrayals appear to treat transgender characters as objects to be exploited rather than the subjects of the story. Henry (2019) noted that many mainstream films display "a cisgender gaze upon transgender bodies and lives, a gaze often focused on the body or physical transition in a mode of voyeuristic spectacle, and marked by curiosity, wariness, pity, or tragedy." Tsai (2010) claimed that mainstream culture exploits "otherness" to make differences more palatable—in this case, making the characters comical (i.e., to not be taken seriously) or psychopathic (i.e., to be viewed as abnormal). In addition, these films reveal a great deal about the current state of politics and community reception, according to Leung (cited in Steinbock, 2019).

History of Gender Variance in US Films

Steinbock (2017) noted that on-screen gender transformation and cross-dressing first appeared in the silent film era (e.g., Charlie Chaplin and Stan Laurel dressing as women). Films such as *I Was a Male War Bride* (1949) and *Some Like It Hot* (1959) used cross-dressing as a comedic device. A cross-dresser is "a person—typically a cisgender man—who sometimes wears feminine clothing in order to have fun, entertain, gain emotional satisfaction, for sexual enjoyment, or to make a political statement about gender roles" ("Gender Identity," n.d.). According to Bornstein and Garber (2008), cross-dressing is more likely theatrical or performance-based rather than an expression of gender identity. The characters in these farces are most often compelled to cross-dress because of desperation or an economic advantage (Miller, 2015). While the endings of the films hint at the possibility that the characters have evolved during their time spent cross-dressing, the lessons are lost once their transgender identities are discarded and the characters resume their cisnormative identities (Miller, 2015).

Films with cross-dressing female leads follow a similar formula, mostly passing as men in order to temporarily gain access to areas deemed off-limits to women (Rigney, 2003). For example, the cisgender female character Yentl dressed as a man and assumed her brother's identity in order to continue her education because females were not allowed to study religious scripture in 1904 Eastern Europe (*Yentl*, 1983). In the film *Albert Nobbs* (2011), Nobbs dons a suit and passes as a man in order to get jobs as a waiter in late-19th-century Dublin. Another character in the film, Hubert Page, similarly takes on the identity of a man after leaving an abusive husband. While some reviews reference Nobbs as transgender, the filmmakers were adamant that Nobbs was not (Advocate, 2011a).

More commonly, cross-dressing films are framed as lighthearted comedies. Set in Paris in 1934, the cisgender female character Victoria, looking to escape poverty, poses as Victor, a female impersonator (*Victor/Victoria*, 1982). In *Shakespeare in Love* (1998), Viola de Lesseps, the daughter of a wealthy merchant, dresses as a man to audition for Shakespeare at a time when all women's roles were played by men. Teen characters also appear in cross-dressing comedies such as *Just One of the Guys* (1985) and *She's the Man* (2006). In *Just One of the Guys*, a male teacher tells high school student Terry that an attractive girl like her should have a backup plan, such as modeling, in case her desired career in journalism falls through. His failure to take her and her writing seriously motivates Terry to cross-dress as a boy and go undercover at a neighboring school with the goal of writing an exposé on how she is treated when others identify her as male. In *She's the Man* (2006), the lead character Viola poses as her twin brother so she can play on the boys' soccer team after her school cuts the girls' squad.

Highly critical of these portrayals, Miller (2015) argued that the characters quickly abandon their disguises in order to resume a cisnormative life. In almost all these films, a heterosexual, cisgender male character falls for the cross-dressing, cisgender female character, adding an element of homophobia that heightens the relief when her true gender is revealed. As with *Yentl*, *Victor/Victoria*, and *Shakespeare in Love*, the audience, as well as the other characters, are assured that the gender transition is temporary by including a big reveal scene (e.g., exposing their womanly breasts). In these examples, gender diversity is purely functional rather than an inherent aspect of their identities.

Perhaps the earliest film to address various aspects of gender variance is Ed Wood's film *Glen or Glenda* (1953). A movie poster described the film as "[t]he strange case of a 'man' who changed his sex!" It portrays gender variations from Patrick/Patricia, who dies by suicide after being arrested a fourth time for dressing as a woman, to Alan/Anne, who is diagnosed as intersex and goes through several operations to present as a woman.

The title character, Glen, is presented as having a compulsion to dress as a woman. The psychiatrist Dr. Alton, also the narrator of the film, explains to Glen that his condition was brought on by the absence of his mother's love and his sister's shunning. He tells Glen that by transferring the need for maternal feelings onto his fiancée Barbara, the compulsion will cease.

A notable feature of transgender films is that they are significantly more likely to focus on transfeminine characters. There is a range of mainstream and indie films, fictional and biographical, spanning the genres of dramas and thrillers to comedies. These films include *The Crying Game*, *Transamerica*, *Normal*, *The Adventures of Priscilla, Queen of the Desert*, *Dressed to Kill*, *Midnight in the Garden of Good and Evil*, *Myra Breckinridge*, *The Danish Girl*, *The World According to Garp*, *Dog Day Afternoon*, *Tangerine*, *Dallas Buyers Club*, *Soldier's Girl*, and *Grilled.* Representations of transgender men have been notably absent in film and television, according to a study by McInroy and Craig (2015). Two non-mainstream comedy films have included prominent transmasculine characters. John Waters's film *Desperate Living* (1977) is an example of a campy portrayal of Mole McHenry, "a man trapped in a woman's body." Mole arrives at the John Hopkins Sexual Reassignment Clinic and threatens the doctor, "If you don't give me a sex change, I'll cut off your peter and sew it on me myself." Mole presents his new penis to his lover, Muffy, who screams, "Get away from me with that deformed worm! You're sick, Mole! You're a weirdo pervert!" She vomits and tells him to rid his body of that "disgusting transplant!" She confesses she only wanted to make Mole jealous by talking about other men. In true Waters form, Mole cuts off the penis with scissors. The main character Anna in *Itty Bitty Titty Committee* (2007) is a lesbian who regrets a one-night stand with Aggie, a transgender man. When Anna questions Aggie's membership in the "CIA," or "Clits in Action," activist group, her friend Sadie responds, "Aggie gets a free pass for being born with a clit."

To date, *Boys Don't Cry* (1999) stands alone as a mainstream box office success featuring a transmasculine character. The film, starring cisgender female actor Hillary Swank, is based on the true story of Brandon Teena. It follows themes common to transfeminine films, such as focusing on surgery/hormones, fear of being outed/rejected by others, and transphobic bullying/violence. The film includes a significant number of transgender tropes, especially in the first 15 minutes. In the opening scene, Brandon is gazing at himself in the mirror as his cousin Lonny cuts his hair to make him look more masculine. Brandon adjusts the roll of socks he has placed in his crotch after Lonny tells him it looks like "a deformity." Lonny also references Brandon's mother's threats to lock him up again for continuing to present as male. Brandon faced obstacles, such as finding and disposing of tampons after getting his period, fearing his gender identity would be revealed. When his girlfriend Lana discovers his chest bindings, he tells her that he is a hermaphrodite. He likewise lies to John and Tom after they find a pamphlet entitled "Cross-dressers and Transsexuals: The Uninvited Dilemma" in his bag. John and Tom take him into the bathroom and pull down his pants to expose his genitalia, and they eventually rape and murder him.

A lesser-known mainstream Hollywood film *3 Generations* (2015) stars cisgender actress El Fanning as Ray, a transitioning boy. Originally titled *About Ray*, Rojas (2017) noted that the film distributor's changing of the title to *3 Generations* "seems to downplay the importance of Ray's situation by comparing his mother's and grandmother's non-existent life crises." While *Boys Don't Cry* took in over $20 million in box office revenue, *3 Generations* only earned around $680,000 (IMDB, n.d.). Fanning is made to look traditionally masculine by adding outward features such as short hair (noticeably a wig), dressing in flannel shirts and stocking caps, and riding a skateboard. The film focuses on predictable themes such as medical transitioning, bullying, and lack of support from family members. The first scene focuses on Ray's doctor explaining hormone treatments. Ray later comes home with a black eye after being confronted by a bully in an alley who asks, "Hey, you a girl or a boy? Huh? Show me your dick, girl." The character Ray laments, "I just want to be normal in a regular school. I get to stop feeling like someone in-between . . . My whole life, I've searched my body for scars because I know part of me is missing." Ray needs his absent father to sign consent forms to start puberty blockers. His father falters, arguing, "What if she changes her mind?" Ray's mother responds, "What if he commits suicide?" Ray's grandmother Dolly, herself a lesbian, tells him, "I just don't understand why we're in such a hurry. I'm sorry, it just feels like mutilation, to me." By the end of the film, Dolly has a change of heart, telling him, "I thought you were too young to know what you wanted, but you do know. And I was just afraid. And now I realize that who you are and who I love is staying the same and everything that's changing is just details . . . I'm saying that it's about time that we had a man in this family."

Television and Media Effects Perspective

Media has been credited as the principal source where both transgender and non-transgender individuals learn about transgender issues (see heinz, 2012; Shelley, 2008). Thus, media representations influence and inform the general public's attitudes and have a significant impact on transgender individuals' gender identity development. Research has shown that media use can help marginalized people feel stronger, fight adversity, and find communities (Craig, McInroy, McCready, & Alaggia, 2015). More specifically,

Capuzza and Spencer (2017) claimed, "Television has the potential to demystify gender nonconformity, to confront transphobia, and to confirm transgender subjectivities" (p. 217). Because viewers' perceptions of transgender characters are mediated by culturally constructed images (Phillips, 2006), an investigation into portrayals of transgender characters is of great importance. Thus, representations shape public opinion and can affect transgender individuals' gender identity development and their lived experiences. Without direct experience with a particular phenomenon, as is often the case with transgender individuals, people receive most of their information through the media (Morgan, Harrison, Chewning, Davis, & Dicorcia, 2007). The importance of this type of analysis cannot be understated. Both transgender and cisgender people turn to the media to learn about transgender matters (McInroy & Craig, 2017); therefore, it is imperative that television producers get it right.

I come at this analysis from a media effects background rather than critical studies. My focus is on audience-centered media effects rather than a critical reading of the text from a cinema studies perspective. For this analysis, I chose to focus on television and streaming series because of their ability to tell more in-depth stories with more screen time than film. Henry (2019) contended that television series (e.g., *Sense8* and *Pose*) have been succeeding over cinema in greater awareness of transgender representation. According to Booth (2015), American audiences learn about its culture from depictions on television and, to a lesser extent, from film. My goal is to research recurring messages that likely create a cultivation effect or sense of normal for the audience. Gerbner (1998) theorized that extended exposure to media, particularly television, produces a cultivation effect that results in television reality becoming more believed and accepted. The increased influence of television is due to its tradition of long-form storytelling. Television has always been a gateway into what it means to be "other" (e.g., Black, gay, etc.). Although gay and lesbian portrayals have become more common place, the absence of transgender representations, particularly transmasculine roles, is stark; therefore, I include social representation analysis.

Making the unfamiliar familiar can be explained using Serge Moscovici's (1973) social representation theory. The theory functions first to establish order that will enable individuals to orient themselves to and master new concepts (Moscovici, 1973). Social representations then create mutually understood categories and definitions within communities, allowing for shared meaning (Moscovici, 1973; Wagner, Universitìt, Duveen, & Gene, 1999). Media, in addition to interpersonal interactions, can shape or create social representations. Sandra Bem referred to media forms as the "cultural transmission" of ways in which humans process information about gender.

Gender schema theory (Bem, 1981) suggests that gender-associated information is understood through a mental framework. In other words, media portrayals can introduce viewers to new ways of thinking about gender.

Another applicable concept is Bandura's social learning theory, where viewers assess punishments and rewards of others when modeling attitudes and behaviors (Bandura, 2001). For example, portrayals presenting characters who are rewarded for subjecting transgender individuals to ridicule or treating them with disdain are more likely to be adopted by viewers. Crime procedurals, which often punish gender-variant characters, casting them as victims or psychotic criminals, send negative messages. Viewers are more likely to adopt positive attitudes toward gender-variant individuals when transgender characters have successful outcomes, such as multiple friends, supportive family members, and romantic partners. In addition, casting transgender actors in these roles can contribute to positive attitude change through increased realism.

Evolution of Transgender Representation

The lack of LGBTQ representation in traditional media (e.g., film and television) is problematic. According to a GLAAD (2020) report on gay, lesbian, bisexual, and transgender representation on television during the 2019–2020 television season, there were just 29 regular and recurring transgender characters on broadcast, cable, and streaming networks (e.g., Netflix, Amazon Prime, Hulu) (Lasky, 2021). The underrepresentation of marginalized communities can lead to what Gerbner and Gross (1976) labeled "symbolic annihilation." In other words, if individuals do not see transgender individuals represented in the media, viewers are less likely to believe that gender variance is legitimate and worthy of protection from harassment and physical harm. Transgender individuals, particularly young people questioning their gender identities, can interpret the absence as an indication that they hardly matter (Kelso, 2015). GLAAD issued a press release stating that the lack of representation marginalizes the transgender communities and is "a missed opportunity by studios and screenwriters to tell fresh stories and better flesh out the worlds they create" (Gouttebroze, 2013).

As with film portrayals, scripted television shows have given significantly more attention to transgender women than transgender men (Ulaby, 2014). Ellis (2020) argued that the lack of transgender men in both entertainment and news media has led to "a cultural perception that they do not exist." In a 2013 study of LGBTQ representation on television, GLAAD found that of the 26 regular and recurring transgender and nonbinary characters on prime-time scripted broadcast TV, only five were transgender men (see Gouttebroze, 2013). By the end of the 2019–2020 season, the number of transgender men had increased to 12 out of 38 transgender characters or 12 out of 882 total characters (Ellis, 2020). Capuzza and Spencer (2017) studied transgender characters who appeared on prime-time scripted television shows from the 2008 through 2014 seasons. Only two of the nine shows featured a transmasculine character. Groundbreaking mainstream television shows that feature significant numbers of transgender characters, most of whom are played by transgender actors, such as *Pose* and *Transparent*, also favor transfeminine characters. Shows featuring ensemble casts of transmasculine characters such as *Brothers* and *Eden's Garden* are often relegated to video-sharing platforms (e.g., YouTube).

According to Adams (2016), "While trans men are spared the worst of our culture's transphobia, our invisibility in the media means America doesn't even know that we exist." When discussing transgender men and the role media plays, Serano (2013) posits that "the media tends to not notice—or to outright ignore—trans men because they are unable to sensationalize them the way they do trans women without bringing masculinity itself into question" (p. 231). According to Dry (2019), Hollywood is still "figuring out what to do with trans male characters." Billard (2016) credited the invisibility of transgender men to the lack of shock or intrigue given to transgender women. In its depictions, television teaches that young transmasculine characters are less scandalous than transfeminine characters, which is understandable given the more acceptable "tomboy" over the "sissy."

Analysis Method

The limited number of transmasculine portrayals must be closely monitored because, as Booth (2011) noted, portrayals can clarify but also risk confusing the viewers. Ringo (2002) further warned that negative depictions could potentially lead to shame for transgender individuals and incite fear among cisgender people. Negative or inaccurate portrayals can offset the positive effects of increased visibility. Even when gender-variant characters are included in fictional media, they are often "poorly written, falling into offensive tropes and stereotypes about transgender people" (Ellis, 2020, p. 30).

This book addresses the unique perspective that television series brings to transgender characters, nearly all of whom are played by actors who identify as transmasculine or nonbinary. I conducted content and textual analyses to highlight examples from television series that potentially influence how viewers see gender variance. I focused on issues facing transgender television characters who were AFAB and now self-identify or are identified by the show (e.g., interviews with producers, promotional materials) as either transmasculine or nonbinary. Since the introduction of Paul Millander, a serial killer on *CSI: Crime Scene Investigation* (2000), and Max on *The L Word* (2006), the number of transmasculine characters has expanded, in part due to the increase of cable outlets and streaming services.

In order to investigate contemporary social constructions of gender-variant characters who were AFAB, I analyzed portrayals of television characters who self-identified and live openly as transgender. I conducted a conventional content analysis where coding categories were formed directly from the text (Hsieh & Shannon, 2005). The goal of the analysis is to provide intricate descriptions of the encoded messages in the text with a focus on themes and patterns that create shared meaning derived from social representation (see Kellner, 1995). After multiple intensive viewings of dialogue and behaviors, I gained a better understanding of individual qualities of plotlines, the transmasculine characters, and their relationships with other characters. I noted evolving narratives and more nuanced treatment of transgender individuals over the past decade, paralleling real-life advances in understanding and acceptance.

Sample

The pool of shows under investigation aired from 2000 to 2021. Television series included in the sample initially aired or were available on broadcast networks, basic cable, premium cable, and popular streaming services, such as Amazon Prime, Hulu, and Netflix. To find relevant examples, I consulted GLAAD's "Where We Are on TV" annual reports. In addition, I searched internet sites for references to transgender characters (e.g., IMDB). In order to keep the sample manageable and keep the focus on shows most likely viewed by large audiences, I excluded more obscure offerings, such as web series or shows only available on video-sharing platforms, such as YouTube.

To be considered, characters must have been major or at least substantial minor characters who appeared in a minimum of three episodes of the series. I relied on direct observations and IMDB listings for episodes. In addition, characters needed to have multiple lines of dialogue and play a significant role in at least one of the show's storylines. I avoided marginal outsiders or guest stars that were only brought in for an "issue-related" plotline, as described by Ulaby (2014). Characters needed to self-identify as transgender or be recognized by the shows' producers and writers as transgender, nonbinary, or gender-questioning; however, it needed to be clear that the character had been AFAB and currently does not identify as cisgender female. I also eliminated cisgender male characters played by transmasculine actors (e.g., Chella Man in *Titans*; Chaz Bono in *American Horror Story*, Elliot Fletcher in *Tell Me Your Secrets*, Michael D. Cohen in Nickelodeon's series *Henry Danger* and *Danger Force*, and Emmett Preciado in *Good Trouble*) and characters in a limited number of episodes (e.g., Tony in *Orphan Black*). The final tally came to 44 characters from 38 series (see Appendix B). Lastly, actors' gender identification was determined mainly through interviews in magazines or online publications where the actors explicitly stated their gender identification (e.g., transmasculine, AFAB nonbinary) and/or preferred pronouns (e.g., he/him/his, they/them/theirs).

2 The Importance of Standpoint

Great care needs to be taken to not only make sure gender-diverse stories are told but that they are told accurately. Even if depictions of transgender characters are not sensationalized, they can still be problematic. According to Serano (2007), "Other depictions are not intended to be blatantly demeaning, yet they still have a drastic negative impact on the lives of transsexuals because the depictions frame transsexuality in terms of non-transgender people's assumptions and interests." Activist Aria Ehren (2015) argued that LGBTQ stories and struggles are being co-opted to appeal to a wide audience. Thus, it is important to allow transgender individuals to tell their own stories in front of and behind the camera. Without their involvement, Ehren cautions the portrayals will likely be inaccurate, and the narratives will be "cleaned up and re-framed" by mainstream media. Henry (2019) lamented the lack of representation behind the camera, stating, "Activism on these issues has played a role in the shifting emphasis from trans people as objects of representation, to the agential opportunities and enterprise trans people have—and want to create—as filmmakers." As transgender comedian Ian Harvie put it, "If you're not at the table, then you're on the menu. That's to say, if you're not included in that process, then you're probably being objectified. If you are included, you're probably being humanized" (cited in Lambert, 2016). This book addresses television shows' attempts to create accurate portrayals by hiring transgender staff, or at a minimum including consultants, and casting transgender actors in the roles whenever possible.

One mission of accurate representation is to incorporate the perspective of transgender individuals. Originating from feminist criticism (see Harding, 2004), standpoint theory scholars argue that knowledge stems from a social position and political experiences. Halpern (2019) explained that "those who are outside of the dominant perspective have access to knowledge that those within it do not." Perspectives outside the power structure offer a privileged position from which "to better see the knowledge and the systems in

DOI: 10.4324/9781003204404-2

which it was created." Thus, "standpoint" influences how people understand themselves and communicate with others, especially when coming from a minority group that lacks power and connections. According to Bowell (n.d.), standpoint theory "asks more from us than just simple perspective-taking, by promoting special consideration for how marginalization may provide more clarity on issues that concern us." Beyond accurate portrayals, media producers have a social responsibility to advocate for the rights and acceptance of those underrepresented (Halpern, 2019), which is best done by inviting them into the process.

Joey Soloway (2018) describes the goal of their work as "lifting and celebrating marginalized voices." Soloway, the creator of *Transparent*, came out as nonbinary after filming the second season. They brought on transgender filmmaker Rhys Ernst and transgender activist Silas Howard to produce and direct episodes. Ernst noted inclusivity on set from always having gender-neutral bathrooms to a cast and crew who were "well-versed" in transgender issues, including gender-neutral pronouns and other etiquettes (cited in McDonald, 2015).

Producers' Backgrounds

It is important who gets to tell which stories and how they get to tell them. In this chapter, I explore the makeup of producers/writers/consultants and actors in groundbreaking shows, as well as their backgrounds and articulated motivations. Rather than conduct interviews for the book, I used information retrieved from secondary sources and popular press interviews that are as easily accessible to lay audiences as media scholars.

At issue is that portrayals of transgender characters are often concentrated in a few shows with some of the same producers. According to GLAAD's annual report for the 2020–2021 television season, nearly one in every five LGBTQ characters appeared on series tied to either Shonda Rhimes or "out" power players, such as Ryan Murphy, Greg Berlanti, and Lena Waithe (see Lasky, 2021; Mitovich, 2021). Although not an example of transmasculine characters, *The Chi* creator, Lena Waithe, introduced the show's first transgender character.

Ryan Murphy's series *Pose*, winner of the GLAAD Media Award for Outstanding Drama Series in 2019 and 2020, featured the largest cast of transgender actors in television history (Real, 2018), as well as the most trans actors of color. Murphy's earlier works, while including transgender characters, were criticized for their portrayals (see Mey, 2015). One of several transgender characters on *Nip/Tuck*, Ava Moore, was depicted as mentally unstable and having an incestuous affair with her adopted teenage son. There were also criticisms from the transgender community about how Murphy handled two characters on *Glee*: Unique and Coach Beiste. Mey (2015) argued that these transgender characters were continually the butt of jokes and portrayed in a way that may perpetuate harmful stereotypes. Murphy more recently stated, "I think the day and age where you put a wig on a straight white man and say he's trans is over" (Real, 2018). There has been an apparent shift in how Murphy portrays and casts transgender characters in his more recent shows. Murphy called his show *Pose* "the highlight of my career . . . [It] will change the lives of so many young kids being able to watch that show" (cited in Chuba, 2018). Murphy stated that he embraces the concept of "show running as advocacy," attributing his passion for telling stories of marginalized groups to growing up gay in a small town in Indiana (Real, 2018).

Murphy hired transgender writer/producers Janet Mock and Our Lady J for *Pose*, "which gave a valuable perspective of the characters' experiences in the show" (Real, 2018). Brad Falchuk, a cisgender heterosexual man who often works with Murphy, stated, "The only way to have compassion is to understand [people's] lives . . . to hear their stories." According to Mock, "A lot of writers in Hollywood believe they can write anything, but Brad understands that we are the authorities on the specific experiences that we go through. He can listen in the room and he can translate the themes and the points of injustice that I faced, as a transgender woman of color, into the character" (Bhattacharji, 2019). *Pose* co-creator Steven Canals, who identifies as queer, added, "How can we tell a story about the ballroom community and transgender people of color and not have them as part of the storytelling process? It was important for us to have consultants be part of the writing process and the production. It makes for a more authentic story" (cited in Nichols, 2018). Lena Waithe, an African American lesbian writer, producer, and actor, emphasized her support for giving voice to the Black LGBTQ community. She is driven to help build a space where intersectional minority groups can continue to tell their stories (Oliver, 2020).

Greg Berlanti, GLAAD Vanguard Award recipient in 2018, created and produced groundbreaking shows with the first transgender recurring character (*Dirty Sexy Money*, 2007) and the first transgender superhero on television (*Supergirl*, 2018) (Boucher, 2019). In addition, he included trans-masculine characters in *The Red Line* and *Chilling Adventures of Sabrina*. Berlanti, who identifies as a gay, cisgender man, spoke out about wanting the stories he was telling to reflect the real experiences of those of various races, genders, and sexualities (cited in Boucher, 2019).

Although Shonda Rhimes identifies as a cisgender, heterosexual woman, she believes everyone should get to see themselves represented on television (cited in Montes, 2012). One of her most popular shows *Grey's Anatomy* included episodes of a transgender teen getting chest masculinization surgery (2013), a two-episode arc (2018) about a doctor who comes in for vaginoplasty surgery, and a nonbinary patient who suffers injuries after a snowmobile accident (2019). In 2017, Alex Blue Davis was added to the cast, a transgender male actor who played transgender male doctor Casey Parker. E. R. Fightmaster, who identifies as nonbinary, was introduced as a nonbinary neuroscientist in season 18 (2021).

One of the goals of *The Fosters*, according to openly gay, cisgender creators Bradley Bredeweg and Peter Paige, was to "open hearts and minds to equality and social issues" (Valenza, 2014). The show won the GLAAD Media Award for Outstanding Drama Series in 2014 and 2016. Notably, they cast transgender actors Tom Phelan in 2014 and Elliot Fletcher in 2016 to play transgender male characters. According to Phelan, there was nothing in the script that was inaccurate (Molloy, 2014). Fletcher reported that the writers were always respectful and open to his feedback, which reflected on his own coming out experience as a transgender man (Henderson, 2018). Bredeweg and Paige later spun off *The Fosters* to *Good Trouble* (2019), which includes multiple transgender and nonbinary characters.

Council of Dads creators Tony Phelan and Joan Rater drew on elements from their own family (their transgender son Tom Phelan played Cole on *The Fosters*) to create the transgender character JJ, played by transgender actor Blue Chapman. They stated, "We're committed to showing something you rarely see on network TV—a family loving their transgender kid" (GLAAD, 2020). According to Jenn Chapman, Blue's mother, "the story and writing was so beautiful, gentle, real, and uplifting. How refreshing it was to see a trans kid loved and supported by his family like we love and support Blue." Because the show's creators have a transgender son, she felt at ease and that the writing would also be sensitive and storylines genuine (GLAAD, 2020).

Work in Progress was created by Abby McEnany, who identifies as a "queer dyke," along with Tim Mason, a straight, cisgender man. According to McEnany, "The reaction was always very *weird*. Like, we're going to bring this straight white cis guy in for *this*?" (Metz, 2019). Transgender filmmaker Lilly Wachowski, one of the show's executive producers, calls Mason a "great ally and he's doing his best to amplify voices and that's what you really need from cis people and straight white guys—listen and amplify marginalized voices."

These producers make up a small number of behind-the-scenes talent, however. A recent viral hashtag #ShowUsYourRoom asked showrunners to take photos of their writers' rooms and post them to social media. Created by Amanda Idoko, the goal of the hashtag was to put pressure on those in charge of hiring and increase "productions with publicly stated diversity initiatives" (Turchiano, 2018). Issues of inaccurate representation arise, as in the case of the film *3 Generations* (2015). Rojas (2017) criticized the director Gaby Dellal for not only casting Elle Fanning, a cisgender female actor, as the transmasculine character, Ray, but also for her lack of understanding of the transgender experience and not going "deeper than headline news stories about trans youth" (Zuckerman, 2015).

When considering the earliest television show portrayals of transmasculine characters, such as *Degrassi: The Next Generation*, it is apparent how far portrayals have come. Michael Grassi (cited in Xtra, 2010) stated that writers for *Degrassi* viewed YouTube video diaries of transgender youth in preparation for their first gender-diverse character, Adam. In an interview with cisgender female actress Jordan Todosey, she described playing Adam as follows: "It was so nice and refreshing to be able to not wear a lot of make-up . . . not caring about all the fashion, glamour." She explained that in playing the role, she had to "keep her hips straight and not do anything 'girly'" (Xtra, 2010). Not to be too critical of this simplistic view of what it means to be transgender, one must consider her age and inexperience and that she played the role back in 2010–2013.

When shows lack a diverse staff, cisgender producers and writers often consult with GLAAD, particularly Nick Adams, the director of transgender media and representation. For example, Jenna Bans (creator of *Good Girls*) and her writers worked with GLAAD to ensure they took a thoughtful approach to the subject of Ben's gender identity (Garrett, 2019). Adams also worked with NBC's high school musical drama *Rise* (Friedland, 2018). Adams gave significant feedback on the dialogue on *The Fosters* "to make it more authentic," according to Henderson (2018). According to Carter Covington, executive producer for *Faking It*, GLAAD helped select the wording of the conversation when Noah came out to Shane, with the goal of modeling "conversations that people have had in real life" (Mackie, 2016). The series *Mistresses* enlisted GLAAD to not only consult on the script but also to help advise the cast and crew on working with the transgender actor Ian Harvie (Lambert, 2016). *Grey's Anatomy* showrunner Krista Vernoff, who describes herself as "only an ally and not a member of LGBTQ community," stated that she worked closely with transgender actor Alex Blue Davis and GLAAD on Casey's storyline (cited in Goldberg, 2018).

Adams encouraged shows to do more to create culturally sensitive writers' rooms, such as making social media managers aware of "proper pronoun usage" (cited in Friedland, 2018). *Star Trek Discovery* executive producer and co-showrunner Alex Kurtzman, along with the show's writers, worked not only to reflect nonbinary actor Blu Del Barrio and transgender actor Ian Alexander's experiences into the show but also to create a safe and healthy work environment for them. Kurtzman noted that *Star Trek* creator Gene Roddenberry's core value was diversity. "Part of the joy of *Star Trek*, especially given the state of the world now, is that we get to create the world that we want to see" (cited in Vary, 2020). Del Barrio explained that they felt wholeheartedly accepted and validated by the staff when they came out as nonbinary. "When I went to our costume department and sheepishly asked them if I could use a binder under my costumes, they went and made me one" (cited in Adams, 2020).

Casting Transgender Characters

There has been much debate back and forth about casting transgender roles; however, as recommended by an earlier reviewer of the book, I do not want this to be a simplistic critique of cis actors taking roles from transgender actors. On the other hand, it would be a conspicuous omission if not covered at all.

Several cisgender actors (compared to zero openly transgender actors to date) have been rewarded for their work as fictional transgender characters in film. For example, Eddie Redmayne won the Oscar for Best Actor for *The Danish Girl* (2016), and Jared Leto won the Oscar for Best Supporting Actor for *Dallas Buyers Club* (2014). *The Crying Game* (1993) received a best supporting actor nomination for Jaye Davidson, while Felicity Huffman won a Golden Globe and received a nomination for an Academy Award for *Transamerica* (2006). Cisgender men and women have also been rewarded for their roles as cross-dressers—for example, Jack Lemmon's Best Actor Oscar nomination for *Some Like it Hot* (1960), Dustin Hoffman's Best Actor Oscar win for *Tootsie* (1983), and Robin Williams's Best Actor Golden Globe win for *Mrs. Doubtfire* (1994). The film *Yentl* won Barbra Streisand, who also starred in the film, the Best Director Golden Globe, the first (and to date the only) woman to win the award (1984). Julie Andrews won the Best Actress Golden Globe for her role in the cross-dressing farce *Victor/Victoria* (1983). Gwyneth Paltrow won the Best Actress Oscar for *Shakespeare in Love* (1999). Glenn Close received a Best Actress Oscar nomination for *Albert Nobbs* (2012). The sole nomination and award for playing a transgender man to date has been for cisgender actress Hillary Swank's Best Actress Oscar for *Boys Don't Cry* (2000).

Many producers have come under fire more recently for their casting of transgender characters and the perceived lack of credibility by critics. Two notable examples of cisgender actresses pulling out of films after being cast in transgender roles are Scarlett Johansson and Halle Berry. Johansson withdrew from the film *Rub and Tug* after her casting generated a backlash from LGBTQ groups (Stedman, 2018). Berry backed out of a potential role as a transgender character after she angered many activists by using incorrect pronouns for the character and describing the plot of the film as "where a woman is transgender" (Jackson, 2020). Activist Serena Daniari (cited in

Jackson, 2020) tweeted, "It absolutely is NOT a female story, it is a story about a man. And why is the aspect of physical transition the focal point for her? Cis peoples' understanding of trans issues is really myopic. Girl watch Disclosure on Netflix." Berry issued a statement via Twitter apologizing for her remarks: "The transgender community should undeniably have the opportunity to tell their own stories" (cited in Jackson, 2020).

As for transgender television roles, Jeffrey Tambor won the Emmy for Outstanding Lead Actor in a Comedy Series for *Transparent* twice (2015 and 2016). Since then, there appears to be an increased appreciation for transgender actors playing transgender characters. For example, nonbinary actor Asia Kate Dillon was nominated as best supporting actor in a drama series for *Billions* at the Critics' Choice Awards in 2017, 2018, and 2019 (although they are now advocating for gender-neutral acting categories). In 2021, Mj Rodriguez became the first openly transgender actor to receive an Emmy nomination for lead acting for her role in *Pose*. While film producers cite the need to cast big-name celebrities and well-known actors, who are almost exclusively cisgender, in order to bring in big box office numbers, television and streaming services do not have those same constraints. One important factor to note is that only eight of the 44 (approximately 20%) transgender and nonbinary recurring or main characters in my sample were played by cisgender actors, with the last one cast in 2018.

Some casting agents argue for selecting the best actor regardless of identification or personal experience, what Booth (2015) describes as the very nature of acting, which is "playing a character unlike oneself." *Degrassi* writer Michael Grassi (cited in Xtra, 2010) admits the show thought about getting a transgender actor to play the role of Adam. He claims they wanted to explore the transitioning and were "just looking for the best person to play the role." Transgender activist Riki Wilchins defended director Kimberly Peirce's casting of Hilary Swank in *Boys Don't Cry*, stating that "it's not fair to go back and apply standards 20 years later that didn't exist back then" (cited in McCabe, 2019). Peirce noted that she assumed she would cast a queer or transgender person; however, she was swayed by Hilary Swank's audition (cited in King, 2019). Rhys Ernst considers casting for transgender roles more complicated than biological determination. He notes that as a transgender director, he might cast a cisgender actor to play a "socially transitioning or pre-transition character" (cited in heinz, 2016, p. 227). Before they came out as nonbinary, Daisy Eagan checked in with the show *Good Trouble*'s producers to see if there would be an issue with their playing a nonbinary character while identifying as cisgender at the time. Eagan reported that "since the character was evolving, the feeling was that it was okay and the representation was fine" (cited in Bastidas, 2019).

Nick Adams (2016), on the other hand, argued that casting cisgender actors send the message that being transgender is an act or a performance. He added putting a man in a dress is "yet another painful reminder that, in the eyes of so many people, transgender women are really just men." Stryker (2008) noted, "Casting particularly well-known cis actors in trans roles helps perpetuate the idea that transness is a kind of deception and that really underneath it all, we're really just cis people in drag." In a review of *The L Word*, Burns (2019) criticized the show's attempt to transform the nonbinary actor Daniela Sea who plays Max into a transgender man post-testosterone, describing the "fake beard pasted on" as almost comical.

Transgender actors delivered even harsher criticism. Trace Lysette, a transgender actress on *Transparent*, tweeted, "[N]ot only do you play us and steal our narrative and our opportunity but you pat yourselves on the back with trophies and accolades for mimicking what we have lived" (cited in Stedman, 2018). Jamie Clayton, a transgender actress on *Sense8*, pointed out that transgender actors are most often limited to auditions for roles as transgender characters. She tweeted that the real issue is that transgender actors "can't get in the room" (cited in Stedman, 2018). Elliot Fletcher recounted his experience seeing that Jared Leto was cast as a transgender woman in *Dallas Buyers Club*. "I couldn't watch it because I knew his portrayal and the way he talked about the character in interviews was just so wrong and that he had no idea what he was talking about. That was such a major disappointment because he won an Oscar for it, too" (cited in Whitney, 2017). Ian Alexander argued that cisgender actors have difficulty accurately portraying transgender characters because they have never experienced gender dysphoria themselves. "Since you pull from your own experiences as an actor, they would never be able to do it with accuracy" (cited in Cuby, 2019).

Pose supervising producer Our Lady J, who cast a record number of transgender actors, pushed back against casting directors who use the excuse that there is not enough talent (Dry, 2019). Co-creator Steven Canals added it was essential and important that they had transgender women of color playing transgender women of color not only for "authentic casting" (Nichols, 2018) but because this community is offered so few opportunities and are "desperate to be a part of Hollywood and a mainstream project" (Real, 2018). Ehren (2015) pointed to the number of transgender actors who are impoverished and underemployed, while cisgender actors who play transgender characters are "praised for their bravery, rewarded for their courage, and passed large paycheques."

Sometimes casting a transgender actor can change the trajectory of a show. In the show *Good Girls*, Ben's character was changed to match the gender identity of the actor. According to Garrett (2019), after casting Isaiah Stannard, who identifies as a transgender male in the role, the show's creator Jenna Bans switched the storyline to make the character Ben transgender as well. E. F. Fightmaster's character Em's pronouns switched from she/her in the second season of *Shrill* to they/them in the third to reflect Fightmaster's nonbinary identity. In the past, GLAAD has worked with the Casting Society of America (CSA) to help increase the number of transgender actors that are seen by casting directors (Adams, 2020). Jen Richards goes on auditions to encourage casting directors, who might not be consciously discriminating against transgender actors, to consider them for roles (cited in Lang, 2019a). JayR Tinaco's management team likewise encourages producers to "switch it up" and cast nonbinary actors like Tinaco (Lang, 2019b).

Besides looking at the negative aspects of casting cisgender actors to play transgender characters, there is added benefit to casting transgender actors in the roles. Kornhaber (2016) argues that trans casting can "humanize a cliché and bring visibility." According to Lang (2019a), "Allowing trans people to play everything from a helicopter pilot to Barista No. 2 sends a powerful message. It says that they are part of the everyday fabric of society, just like everyone else." The casting of a transgender individual in *The Fosters* to fill the role of Cole carried with it an opportunity to educate the public (Molloy, 2014). In the beach scene, Phelan's chest masculinization surgery scars were a sign that his gender identity was not temporary or a disguise. Nick Adams (2016) contends,

> When you hire a trans actor, they don't have to spend weeks or months 'preparing and researching' to play a trans person. They can walk in the door on day one, ready to deliver an authentic, nuanced performance. You get the added bonus of having someone on set who can tell you if something about the dialogue or the characterization is falling into tropes and clichés that will ultimately not reflect well on you or the project.

It is important to note that more and more transgender actors are taking to social media and becoming social justice warriors. Their personal experiences, often muted in traditional film and television stories, are given unedited exposure. Murchison (2017) argued that as more transgender individuals open up and more cisgender people get to know them, the more likely transgender people will gain equality. Ryan Cassata shared on *Larry King Live* that he does not "run down the hall screaming" he is transgender; however, he feels it is important to put a face to the story, to take away the "freakish status." Evie MacDonald, the first transgender actor to play the lead role in an Australian television series (*First Day*), came out when she was nine years old. She uses her social media platforms to advocate for transgender rights and educate people on what being transgender means (CBC, 2021). Without these media examples, young people may think they are the only ones struggling. JayR Tinaco commented, "I remember growing up and not having anyone that I could relate to. It alienates you and for a young kid in a small country town, that can end up being pretty dangerous" (Leighton-Dore, 2019). Brian Michael Smith argued that "the most important thing is to change this perception that trans people are trans before they are people." Exposure to more transgender actors "gives audiences an opportunity to see them as more than just one thing" (Lang, 2019a). Ian Alexander noted, "People have messaged me saying that I helped them come out to their family or helped them to be more confident with their identities" (Villarreal, 2020). According to Tom Phelan, the feedback from *The Fosters* has been overwhelmingly positive. "A lot of kids have been telling me their stories and telling me that it's been great to see someone like them on television" (cited in Palmer, 2015).

As the first transgender contestant on *Dancing with the Stars*, Chaz Bono noted that he used his platform to speak out and help people and personalize an experience people may not understand. Skyler explained that he went "Trans 101" with his appearance on *Queer Eye*: "I'm going to teach some middle-America housewife moms how to care for their transgender kids when they come out by being open and understanding their kids better" (cited in Kaspar, 2018). In 2021, Kade Gottlieb became the first transgender man to compete on *RuPaul's Drag Race*. Performing as Gottmik, she shared that she felt a lot of pressure taking on an activist role; however, RuPaul told her that just being there was enough (cite in Visage, 2021). She added that she is motivated to speak out by the political climate, the murder of transgender people, and homeless LGBTQ youth.

Final Thoughts

Who tells a story has a significant influence on how it is told, particularly the retelling of real-life stories. Diane Middlebrook's (1998) biography *Suits Me: The Double Life of Billy Tipton* received harsh criticism for referring to Tipton as a woman disguised as a man and motivated by career ambitions. Critics charged that Middlebrook, as a cisgender woman, had shown little insight into gender-diverse experiences. In the documentary *No Ordinary Man* (2021), on the other hand, transgender writers and activists such as Amos Mac, Stephan Pennington, and C. Riley Snorton identified Tipton as transgender. The film highlighted the perspective of contemporary transmasculine actors who were speaking in Tipton's voice, as though they were auditioning to play him in the film. As transmasculine actors, Alex Blue Davis, Marquise Vilson, Emmett Preciado, Scott Turner Schofield, Ellis

David Perry, Ryan Cassata, and Carter Ray added their individual interpretations of what life might have been like for Tipton. Zeke Smith, a creative consultant and contributor to the documentary *Disclosure: Trans Lives on Screen* (2020), partnered with GLAAD and Nick Adams to encourage transgender individuals to tell their stories. "Any person who does not see themselves in media, don't expect someone else to do it for you. Write the script. Be an actor. Be a comedian. Be a musician. If your voice is missing, it's because you need to lend it. So do so" (cited in Feder, 2020).

3 Transgender Across Genres

Clark (1969) identified four stages of media representation for social groups, with the first being non-representation or exclusion followed by ridicule, regulation, and respect. When characters do appear on screen, as in stage two, they are often objects of derisive humor. In the third stage, the group is present but in limited ways. The incorporation of characters and their roles in everyday life marks the final stage. There are variations of this journey from ridicule to respect in different television genres. One concerning issue is that when transgender characters are visible, they are often relegated to unflattering representation in limited media genres. In Phillips's (2006) study of films that featured transgender characters, he noted those portrayals were most often classified as comic figures, psycho-trans, or drama queens. A review of television genres gives a better idea of how the industry treats transgender issues depending on the type of shows.

Genre is a powerful driver of texts. It gives the industry a way to market television series to specific audiences. Fictional characters in my sample who appear in a minimum of three episodes appeared in series in drama, comedy, or comedy-drama genres. Additional transgender individuals who appear in the reality genre are also considered in the analysis in order to give a more complete picture of transgender representation on television. An important rationalization for looking at genres is that producers enlist different strategies to entertain and educate according to their ultimate goals. For example, dramas focus on conflict to draw in viewers and increase ratings, comedies select themes to create incongruity or an opportunity for audience members to feel superior, and reality shows capitalize on the novelty of gender diversity.

A consistent theme that emerged from my sample was the treatment of characters depending on if they had an ongoing presence in the series versus appearing in only one or two episodes. Unlike movies with clear beginnings, middles, and ends, serial TV shows allow for multiple beginnings, middles, and ends (Master Class, 2021). According to industry experts, "Each TV script is part of a larger narrative, with multiple character and story arcs

DOI: 10.4324/9781003204404-3

divided across a number of episodes and seasons. TV shows typically focus on the writing rather than the visuals to drive the story. The stories and characters will continue to grow into the next episode—except for episodic series which have standalone format."

Dramas

Merriam-Webster's Dictionary (2021a) defines drama as "a category of narrative fiction (or semi-fiction) intended to be more serious than humorous in tone." The assumption is that television dramas will contain a certain number of conflicts or challenges. Twenty-six out of 38 shows in my sample were dramas (not including the six comedy-dramas). According to *The Screenwriters Taxonomy*, dramas are usually qualified with subgenres labels that indicate a specific setting, subject matter, or tone (Williams, 2018). Subgenres include soap operas, police crime dramas, political or legal dramas, domestic dramas, teen dramas, and comedy-dramas. Most of the subgenres covered in this next section tend to include gender-diverse characters, mainly in one-time appearances that focus on their transness. For example, crime and hospital dramas are set up to have a steady flow of one-episode characters as victims, perpetrators, or patients. I am including some examples of one-time characters, who were outside my sample parameters, for comparison in the following analysis.

Crime Dramas

Criminal procedural shows (e.g., *Bones*, *The Closer*, *CSI: Crime Scene Investigation*, *Law & Order: Special Victims Unit*) have a history of using transgender characters for shock effect and framing gender diversity as dangerous. They are also known to exploit the victimization that transgender individuals experience in real life (particularly *Law & Order: SVU*, which its title insinuates transgender characters as special victims). Halberstam's (2005) description of "destabilizing effects of the queer narrative" in films such as *Psycho* (1960), *Dressed to Kill* (1980), and *Silence of the Lambs* (1991) are also apparent in procedural crime dramas. Many depictions in crime dramas portray transgender individuals as one-dimensional victims, the objects of ridicule or pity, or mentally unstable perpetrators who incite fear. While claiming to increase public awareness of violence against transgender individuals (Shelley, 2008), producers tend to also exploit transgender characters' pain and perpetuate negative stereotypes. GLAAD's (n.d.) analysis of transgender characters on US television series between 2002 and 2012 found that transgender characters were killers or villains in at least 21% of episodes and victims in at least 40%. Even in comedies, transgender or cross-dressing women were portrayed as victims of homicide—for example, Beverly LaSalle on *All in the Family* (1975) and Stephanie on *Ally McBeal* (1997). These roles tend to be played by guest stars; therefore, little or no time is spent focusing on these one-episode characters as people beyond their "transness."

The first recurring transmasculine character in my sample, Paul Millander (*CSI*), is representative of Phillips's (2006) "psycho-trans" character. Millander becomes a serial killer following his mother's rejection after his gender confirmation surgery. The show crams a significant number of transphobic clichés and references to his struggle with his gender identity. Although he appears in a three-episode arc beginning with the pilot of *CSI: Crime Scene Investigation* (2000), it is not until his third episode, "Identity Crisis" (2002), that Millander is revealed to be transgender. In a deadpan tone, forensic entomologist Grissom notes, "Paul killed Pauline, but he didn't murder her." This multi-episode depiction appears to be an outlier. Transgender characters are more likely to appear in a single episode and be portrayed as the victim. In *Cold Case*'s usual style, episode "Boy Crazy" (2007) flashes back to 1963. Sam's father commits him to a psychiatric conversion facility after a bully rips Sam's shirt open and exposes him to the rest of the class as transgender. After failed attempts to force Sam to present as a girl, he is left comatose from electric shock treatment. *Law & Order: SVU* episode "Service" (2018) portrays a more contemporary transgender individual where the character, a military officer, is a witness rather than the victim or perpetrator of a crime. Sargent Jim Preston is reluctant to testify in a rape case against a fellow officer because he fears his gender identity will be exposed and thus risking discharge. After his testimony leads to the conviction of the rapist, dozens of service people in the courtroom stand and salute him as he leaves the courtroom.

The sole gender-diverse character in a lead role in a crime show in my sample appeared in FOX's *Deputy* (2019). The character Bishop, who is the head of the Deputy of Los Angeles' security detail and then later an intelligence expert, comes out as nonbinary in the seventh episode. Their boss and coworkers are very accepting about their coming out, unlike single episodes such as *Cold Case*'s "Boy Crazy" (2007) discussed earlier. The present-day portrayal of gender diversity continues to be less than sensitive, similar to the 1963 flashback scenes. For example, one of the detectives investigating the case calls Sam the victim a "gender-bending girl." Another detective states, "She was a boy, inside of a girl who liked a boy? Making my head hurt."

Hospital/Medical/Rescue Dramas

Hospitals are a prime location for discussions of gender-affirming surgeries and medical aspects of transitioning. These shows also feature a revolving cast of patients and rescue victims. Episodes range from a one-time transgender patient in *Medical Center* (1975) to various transgender characters in Ryan Murphy's series *Nip/Tuck* (2003–2010). Character portrayals can be educational and even inspirational. For example, the medical series *Royal Pains* won a GLAAD Media Awards for Outstanding Individual Episode for a series without a regular LGBTQ character for their treatment of a transgender teen in "The Prince of Nucleotides" (2016).

The series *L.A. Doctors* (1999) features the first scripted transgender male character on television (Anderson, 2015), a portrayal that focuses on his misuse of unprescribed hormones. *Grey's Anatomy* (2013) and *New Amsterdam* (2018) include young patients coming in for chest masculinization surgery. Transgender actor Emmett Preciado plays a transgender man with a rapidly growing brain tumor who discovers he is pregnant in an episode of *The Good Doctor* (2021). The plot focuses on his struggles with the decision to terminate or carry the pregnancy, which also means risking his life and his mental well-being as he will need to stop his testosterone treatments. In a good dramatic fashion, surgery successfully removes the brain tumor, and the pregnancy can continue.

Much like criminal shows, nearly all appearances of transgender characters in hospital dramas are patients who appear in a single episode except for Dr. Casey Parker and Dr. Kai Bartley in *Grey's Anatomy*. In season 14 (2017), transgender actor Alex Blu Davis joined the cast as a first-year intern. His identity is rarely referenced, and his status is not revealed until his fifth episode. Producers took great care to make him more than his gender identification—for example, not including his character in a storyline about a nonbinary patient (Goldberg, 2018). E. R. Fightmaster's character in season 18 is identified as nonbinary with a simple reference to their pronoun in their first appearance. As of 2021, no other mention of their gender identity is mentioned.

Speculative Fiction

Subgenres such as science fiction present opportunities to experiment with different types of characters. Kerry's (2009) analysis of the *Star Trek* franchise demonstrated how the science fiction genre has long created space for gender-diverse characters. Netflix's *Another Life* showrunner Aaron Martin explained, "You would hope that in the future, all these ridiculous things that are supposedly problems in the present—which bathroom to use and the debate around gender and gender identity—that nobody cares" (cited in August, 2019). *Sense8* not only featured transgender actress Jamie Clayton as transgender female Nomi, it was co-created by transgender filmmakers Lana Wachowski and Lilly Wachowski. Apart from her transphobic mother wanting her lobotomized, Nomi was allowed to be a regular character apart from her transness.

Six of the 44 characters who appeared in five out of the 38 shows in the sample came from the speculative fiction genre. In *Chilling Adventures of Sabrina*, Roz's grandmother is a blind mystic seer who recognizes Theo as a young man before he fully understands his own gender identity. Theo is also visited by the spirit of his androgynous Aunt Dorothea, who encourages him to go to the witches for help with his physical transition. Season two of *The OA* explored a different dimension where Buck had not yet socially or medically transitioned and presents as Michelle. The series *Y: The Last Man* (2021), adapted from a DC Comic series, explored a dystopian world where all beings with a Y chromosome have died, including both cisgender and transgender women with a Y chromosome. Elliot Fletcher plays a transgender man named Sam who survives, as do other transgender men without a Y chromosome. The shortage of testosterone, since the pharmacies have all been looted, factors into the plot of the show. Yorick, the only cis man to survive, is mostly mistaken for a transgender man.

Star Trek: Discovery (2020) stands out for featuring two gender-diverse characters, Blu del Barrio as nonbinary character Adira and Ian Alexander as their transgender boyfriend Gray. Gray dies but comes back in holographic form. Hugh promises Gray, "We'll find a way to help you be seen, truly seen by everyone," which is clearly a metaphor for transgender characters being seen. Contrast this sensitive treatment to *Deep Space 9* (1995), where there is a reference to an off-screen male character who is pregnant, or "budding," and the *Enterprise* (2001) episode "Unexpected," which includes a storyline where cismasculine character Commander Tucker becomes the first human male to temporarily host a pregnancy. These instances of playing with gender and male pregnancy tend to be more sensationalistic than advancing acceptance of transgender individuals.

Dramas Conflicts

Most of the recurring characters in my sample come from standard serial dramas, which are unlikely to have single-episode, one-off characters. Recurring television characters appear to be treated with greater respect; however, this is not to say there is no conflict regarding their gender identity. Only four characters appeared to be free of conflict issues associated with their gender as of 2021: Lindsay (*Good Trouble*), Gray (*Discovery*), Kai (*Grey's Anatomy*), and James (*The Politician*). A variety of conflict themes emerged, ranging from misgendering to death threats. Conflicts tended to resolve over time, and disrespectful characters (mostly one-offs) are almost always quickly called out on their behavior and corrected by the transgender character or an ally (mostly recurring). Younger characters occasionally faced bullying; however, those cases were generally resolved, often in the span of a single episode.

There appears to be a conscious effort to avoid slurs, presenting a gentler tone on television in contrast to film. The most egregious examples are heard in episodes of *Degrassi* (2010 and 2011), where at least two different cisgender characters refer to a transmasculine character as a "tranny." The slur also appeared on *The L Word* (2008) and most recently on *Glee* (2015). Another common term is "freak," which is used in *Degrassi* (2010), *The Fosters* (2015), *Dead of Summer* (2016), and *Faking It* (2016). For as crude as the series *Shameless* was, there were surprisingly few derogatory labels or slurs targeting Trevor during his run on the show (2016–2017).

A range of behavioral conflicts is present, from mild and shunning to sexual assault and threats of violence. On the milder yet still harmful side, six-year-old JJ (*Council of Dads*) is disinvited to parties after his parents find out about his gender identity. Max (*The L Word*) has issues regarding his place in the lesbian community after he no longer identifies as a lesbian or a woman. Nonbinary Cal and Layla (*Sex Education*) are forced to comply with gendered school uniforms by an overzealous headteacher. At times, disparagement came in the form of hurtful pranks. Theo (*Chilling Adventures of Sabrina*) opens his locker, and hundreds of pantyliners and tampons fall out. Kevin's (*Charmed*) roommates leave a bra on his bed. Coach Beiste's (*Glee*) car is vandalized with the slur "Tranny." Other times, perpetrators use direct threats and verbal harassment. Drew (*Dead of Summer*) is threatened with being outed, while Star (*David Makes Man*) is threatened with physical harm. Cole (*The Fosters*) is harassed in line for the men's bathroom. Chris (*Work in Progress*) also expresses worries about bathroom safety. Sometimes the harm was inflicted in the past, recounted with few details. Paul (*9-1-1: Lone Star*) reflected that when he was growing up, there were "a lot of folks that wanted to hurt me." Toine (*Queen Sugar*) likewise disclosed he had troubles when he was young. On-screen conflict ranged from a boy throwing food at Ben (*Good Girls*) in the cafeteria, while others laugh, to Michael (*Rise*) being pushed around in *Rise* to Theo's (*Chilling Adventures of Sabrina*) getting a bloody lip.

Other shows include characters recounting how they were sexually assaulted or sexually harassed off-screen, such as peers trying to pull down Ben's (*Good Girls*) pants and pulling up Theo's (*Chilling Adventures of Sabrina*) shirt. On-screen, Bianca rips open Adam's (*Degrassi*) shirt to expose his bindings over his T-shirt. From the playbook of "trans panic" over finding out she is attracted to someone she thinks is cisgender, she threatens, "Touch me again, and I'll kill you." Upon hearing the rumors, the bullies pressure Adam to "whip it out" at the urinal in the boys' restroom.

Adam is thrown against a glass door, which shatters, but he is not seriously hurt. One of the bullies makes a "we are watching you" gesture (i.e., pointing two fingers to his eyes and then at Adam) as he walks away. It is important to note that violent scenes are either described after the fact or not explicitly shown. Even in most television crime procedural dramas, the violence happens off-screen.

Comedies

Insensitive or exploitative examples are not limited to dramas. Comedies include jokes made at the expense of transgender characters. In film, comedies almost exclusively misrepresent gender diversity as cross-dressing, where transformations are portrayed as playful and temporary (Phillips, 2006). Miller (2015) referenced cross-dressing farces with visual jokes, often including a man dressed as a woman teetering in heels, such as the films *Some Like It Hot*, *Tootsie*, and *Mrs. Doubtfire*. Disguise comedies on television include *Ugliest Girl in Town* (1968–1969), *Bosom Buddies* (1980–1982), and *Work It* (2012). Corporal Klinger on *M*A*S*H* (1972–1983) dresses as a woman to get a Section 8 discharge from the Army, showing he is mentally unfit for service.

The masculine version of the cross-dressing trope is rarer; however, two examples can be found on television situation comedies targeted to adolescents. In Nickelodeon's *Zoey 101*, "Girls Will Be Boys" (2005), Lola disguises herself as a boy to prove that boys can still act the same if a girl is around them. To portray her "maleness," she spits and belches in addition to putting on a short-haired wig. She briefly breaks character when she sees a cute blouse on another girl and exclaims how cute it is. Lola is ultimately outed when she is pushed into a swimming pool and loses her wig. In the first episode of Disney Channel's *The Suite Life on Deck*, "The Suite Life Sets Sail" (2008), cisfeminine character Bailey pretends to be a boy so she can attend the ship's boarding school since all of the girls' spots are taken. To disguise her femaleness, Bailey wears baggy clothes and conceals her long hair under a cap. She nearly blows her cover when she inadvertently mentions the need to moisturize. She is eventually outed when she falls in the swimming pool, and she loses her hat. In these examples, the portrayal of gender diversity is purely functional rather than an inherent aspect of their identities.

To help understand the treatment of transgender issues in comedy settings, I organized jokes according to the superiority, relief, and incongruity theories of humor. The following examples are mostly geared toward transgender women in situation comedies. In addition, targets of humor are almost exclusively one-off characters.

Superiority Theory

Superiority humor is based on status differences (Hobbes, 1651/1958). According to Goldstein (1976), the feeling of superiority typically focuses on either the inadequacies of an individual or a deviation from the norm within society. Miller (2015) argued that comedy, the most popular form regarding transgender individuals in film, portrays transgender characters as objects of ridicule. Transgender people are portrayed as psychopaths or inferior freaks to be laughed at. Berger (1993) added that the types of jokes a person enjoys reflect the character of that person and the ethos of a given society.

Joke setups throughout the history of comedy films and television sitcoms include cases where cisgender characters are wronged by what they interpret as deception by the transgender person. To calm the audience's fears of cisgender characters being duped, writers target the transgender characters with jokes since laughter provid[es] "a way of asserting power over terrible threats" (Douglas, 2010, p. 65). Unlike the cross-dressing examples described earlier, transgender characters cannot simply take off a hat or a wig and revert to their gender assigned at birth. When the cisgender character is surprised by the reveal in these portrayals, it taps into a form of "trans panic." A common trope is the one-off character who returns and surprises the main character with the transition reveal, as seen in *The Jeffersons* (1977), *WKRP in Cincinnati* (1980), *Night Court* (1985), *Married . . . with Children* (1994), and *Just Shoot Me* (2000). The cisgender characters feel tricked and become defensive about being made fun of by other characters; therefore, they lash out at the friend who has transitioned. In the context of comedy, effects are more likely humiliation than physical harm to the target. Humor in this regard is a form of superiority where cisgender individuals represent the norm. These jokes degrade not only the individual but the entire group the character represents.

Sepinwall (2019) found anti-transgender dialogue and slurs in many television episodes and storylines. Numerous films and TV shows in recent decades featured cisgender straight men crying (*Californication*, 2012), gargling (*Ally* McBeal, 2000), or vomiting (*The Cleveland Show*, 2009; *Family Guy*, 2010) after learning they had kissed or slept with a transgender woman. These scenes harken back to *Ace Ventura* (1994) type of disparagement humor. *The Connors* (2020) offered a retort to these past transphobia jokes. Becky's boss Robin, who struggles with disclosing her transgender identity, explains, "Movies like *Ace Ventura* where all the men vomit because they find out the woman is transgender, it doesn't make you want to share stuff." Becky responds, "Maybe they were vomiting because they found out they were in *Ace Ventura*."

Even shows that were supposed to be feminist or enlightened have instances of transphobic humor. In *Sex and the City* (2000) episode "Cock-a-Doodle-Do!" transgender sex workers are talking outside Samantha's new apartment. She laments, "I am paying a fortune to live in a neighborhood that's trendy by day and tranny by night." Three times in voice-overs, Carrie uses the expression "half-women" to describe them, such as "Samantha always knew how to get her way with men, even if they were half-women." Lavern Cox (cited in Schneider, 2019) later commented, "It was disappointing to me, as a black trans woman, to see black trans women enter the world of 'Sex and the City' and be so thoroughly othered." Schneider (2019) cites a warning of "reactionary woke analyses" or looking back at past episodes through today's lens.

Ally McBeal included two transgender storylines: Stephanie in 1997 and Cindy in 2000. While Richard, one of the law firm's partners, is a notorious bigot, Ally makes some slips for cheap laughs even though she is supposed to be an enlightened feminist. Stephanie, showing off a dress she has sewn, asks Ally, "Won't I make a beautiful bride? Now, if I can only latch onto a husband." Without thinking, Ally responds, "Well, if you go to prison, you'll have plenty of time to be a wife. Oh my god. I have a way with Freudian slips." Stephanie takes her comment in stride: "So do I. I'm wearing one." One of Ally's coworkers, Mark, begins to date Cindy, whom he thinks is a cisgender woman. Ally again makes a slip about Cindy, telling Mark, "There might be circumcisions you don't know about. Circumstances."

In contrast to one-appearance or minor transgender characters, Alexis is a major character in *Ugly Betty* (2007–2008). Played by cisgender actress Rebecca Romijn, Alexis returns to her family's publishing empire as a transgender woman after gender confirmation surgery. Wilhelmina has a packet of photos spanning the transformation of Alexis and drops a one-liner, "Now you see it. Now you don't." Other references are not so subtle. Lawyer Grace Chin tells Alexis, "You don't need a lawyer, you need a good shrink, and maybe a closer shave." In another exchange, Alexis becomes the aggressor. "I have much bigger dreams [than the magazine]." Her brother Daniel jokes, "Like what? A uterus?" Alexis gets the last laugh: "You can say it, but can you spell it?"

Relief Theories

Relief or release humor involves the reduction of psychological tension (see Berlyne, 1972). Freudian in nature, jokes can focus on genitalia (Freud, 1928) or a relief from political correctness, both of which are often related to transgender subjects. For example, in a *Two and a Half Men* (2013) storyline,

Alan dates a transgender woman Paula. She describes her surgical transition as starting with having her penis cut in half. Seeing Alan cringe, she adds, "I'll spare you what happened to my balls." Alan jokes, "I know what just happened to mine." Later at the movie theater's concession stand, Alan asks Paula, "Do you want to split a hotdog? Oh, I am so sorry!" As Alan debates whether to continue seeing her, he reasons, "I'm not going to let one little thing come between us." Paula replies, "Oh, it wasn't little," to which Alan responds, "A little bit of dating advice, no guy likes to hear that his girlfriend had a bigger penis than he does." *Sex and the City* (2000), in the same episode discussed earlier, Samantha invites the transgender women over for a cookout. Samantha picks up a hotdog and asks, "Who wants a wiener?" One of the guests responds, "Girl, I'm trying to get rid of one of them!"

Jokes about transgender men target adding a penis or testicles rather than removing them. In an episode of *Golden Girls* (1987) where a transgender man revealed his gender identity, Rose asks naively, "What about the parts they put on? Do they test them first?" Dorothy responds sarcastically, "Of course, Rose. Like windshield wipers." Rose then asks, "What are they made of?" Dorothy, who is losing patience with Rose's naïveté, answers, "Silly Putty, Rose!" In an earlier transgender storyline on *Two and a Half Men* (2003), Charlie tells his former girlfriend, who is now a transgender man, "Nice to see you again. Good luck with the penis." Charlie is later concerned that having dated a transgender man pre-transition makes him gay. I could only find one joke about a transmasculine character on *Pose*, a show that is focused overwhelmingly on transgender women. In a cameo appearance, Laith Ashley plays Sebastian, who straddles Candy, much to her delight. She squeals, "I love me a man in any form. Whoo! I don't care how they started out as long as he ends up on top of me."

Incongruity Theory

This theory is sometimes referred to as incongruity-resolution theory. Morreall (1983) explained that humor involves "something that violates our mental patterns and expectations." Veatch (1998) added, "[T]he perceived situation is seen as normal, and where, simultaneously, some affective commitment of the perceiver to the way something in the situation ought to be is violated." This type of humor may present a less hurtful tone in that it can distract or deflect disparagement away from the expected target. Jokes sometimes emphasize misunderstandings rather than target the transgender character. For example, in *All in the Family* (1975), Beverly LaSalle introduces herself as a transvestite. Misunderstanding the term "transvestite," Edith responds, "You sure fooled me. You don't have an accent at all." When Paula (*Two and a Half Men*, 2013) first discloses to Alan that for the first 40 years of her life, she was a man named Paul, Alan nervously responds, "Wow . . . You don't look . . . 40."

In *One Day at a Time* (2018), Elena informs her grandmother, "Some people are gender non-conforming, they have preferred pronouns." Lydia, thinking she said "pronounce," replies in her thick Cuban accent, "Ah! I am Lydia. Pronounced 'Ly-dee-a.'" In the same episode of *Golden Girls* (1987) mentioned before, Gil Gessler is a shy, mild-mannered man running for city council. Gil confesses that he was previously a housewife named Anna Maria Bonaduce. Suspicious that there was something about him, Sophia tells Dorothy, "Five more minutes, I would have had it." Dorothy responds, "Ma, how could you know? No one knew." Sophia replies, "Please, look at his nose. Of course, he's Italian." These jokes play on misunderstanding words and or pointing to incongruous situations to create humor that is less disparaging and, quite honestly, funnier.

Satire

Satire and mocking the status quo are often tools used to disarm prejudice. The comedy sketch show *Portlandia* is known for its gender-bending characters, such as Candace (played by Fred Armisen), from the feminist bookstore sketch. In one episode, Candace lectures her son Bob about not recognizing gender. Bob notes, "I just feel like I'm good at recognizing a woman when I see one." Candace challenges him, "How? What are you? Are you a detective? A gender detective? Lifting up skirts and pulling down pants, getting in there with your magnifying glass?" Candace later adds, "I'm proud of you, even though you are a man." While Bob claims he can't change that, Candace's partner Toni notes that he actually can. Bob, giving up, replies, "I know. I probably won't this late in the game."

In reaction to the sketch, Portland's In Other Words bookstore released the following statement criticizing the show as "trans-antagonistic" and "trans-misogynist." "Fred Armisen in a wig and a dress is a deeply shitty joke whose sole punchline throws trans femmes under the bus by holding up their gender presentation for mockery and ridicule" (cited in Fitzpatrick, 2016). Thomson (2017) defended the show responding, "By no means are the altered voices or drag performances meant to be interpreted as an attack on transgendered people or drag performers like some believe. Instead, the show hyperbolizes and criticizes the gender binaries that our society has created." She added, "The show's use of humour entertains audiences and helps to engage them in the incredibly informative and valuable messages being explored."

Another example of satire is from the always irreverent *South Park*. The series features a teacher Mr. Garrison, who, after nine seasons, transitions to a woman in "Mr. Garrison's Fancy New Vagina" (2005). Later, in the episode "Eek, A Penis!" (2008), Mr. Garrison transitions back to a man. As a spoof, the surgeon performs "negroplasty" to make Kyle African American so he can dunk a basketball and "dolphinoplasty" to surgically alter Kyle's father's appearance to resemble that of a dolphin. *One Day at a Time* (2018) introduces and yet slightly mocked the use of preferred pronouns. As Elena's friends share their names and preferred pronouns, Elena's mother responds, "I'm Penelope. My thoughts are 'Huh?' and 'What?' Seriously, what is happening?" A round of "who's on first" type of dialogue ensues.

LYDIA: Don't worry. I'll be watching them.
ELENA: Why would you be watching Syd? [Syd uses "they/them" pronouns.]
LYDIA: I meant you.
ELENA: My pronoun is "her."
LYDIA: I thought [Dani] was "her."
ELENA: We're both "her."
PENELOPE: You meant them.
ELENA (pointing to Syd): No, "they is them." Stop making this confusing!

A cisgender character Dr. Berkowitz, who has been listening in the background, responds to Elena's brother, "What a nice group of . . . human people friends. [Whispering] I heard about the pronoun thing. Now I'm terrified to speak." The whole scenario comes off as more of a gag than a respectful treatment of preferred pronouns.

Humor and Recurring Characters

In my sample, the comedy shows with recurring gender-diverse characters are split between the traditional half-hour comedies *Transparent*, *Faking It*, *House of Lies*, *One Day at a Time*, *Shrill*, and *Work in Progress* and the full-hour comedy-dramas *Glee*, *Good Girls*, *Better Things*, *Shameless*, *The Politician*, and *Sex Education*. Recurring characters offer a different tone since the relationships between characters are more developed and involve few if any traditional jokes. The following examples of humor that reference transgender individuals are more subtle than standard setup-punchline jokes. Multi-camera sitcoms have the expectation of punchlines and, since they are filmed in front of a live studio audience, often add in extra laugh tracks. These types of sitcoms were represented in the earlier analysis of humor theory. The shows in my sample with recurring transgender male characters happened to be all single-camera comedies, which appear more like film. Writers can take their time with humor since the expectation of a joke every few minutes/seconds is not part of the formula.

When Alice (*Good Trouble*) reveals that Lindsay now goes by "they/them," Sydney, a cisgender character, responds, "There's a lot of that going around." Noticing that she is coming across as intolerant, she continues, "Which I fully support." In order to lighten the mood, she jokingly adds, "It's just tough to remember. Life is so hard for a white woman." *Work in Progress* also uses this tactic to relieve tension. The series features among its cast Julia Sweeney playing a version of herself. She is mostly known for her *Saturday Night Live* character Pat. Pat is a gender-ambiguous character who causes discomfort in others because they cannot identify Pat's gender. After Chris watched some clips, he tells Julia, "I don't mean to be rude, but Pat was not exactly a positive portrayal for gender nonconforming folks . . . Honestly, the most offensive thing to me were those khakis." They all laugh, even Abby, who is a masculine-presenting woman, was traumatized by Pat.

In an episode of *Shameless*, Ian has the following discussion with Kevin about having sex with Trevor. There is not so much a joke here as a humorous tone to the dialogue, focusing on Ian and Kevin's lack of understanding.

IAN: He has a vagina.
KEVIN: Like a real live vagina or he acts like a pussy?
IAN: It's a real live vagina but I'm not supposed to call it that because it's a nonfactor.
KEVIN: So, is it imaginary?
IAN: No, it's more like a man cave.

In another scene, Taylor (*Billions*) gets a large flower arrangement from an admirer delivered to the office. Bill responds, "Nice weeds. So, this guy or girl or whatever couldn't spring for roses?" Mafee, stereotyping both lesbians and hypermasculine men, adds, "I'd have gotten you a K. D. Lang album and tickets to UFC, cover all the bases." While these jokes rely on stereotypical comments about cisgender men and lesbians, Taylor, who is nonbinary, appears to take the comments in stride.

9-1-1: Lonestar presents a humorous scene meant to expose a racist older woman who keeps calling the police on her Latinx neighbors. When the police go to arrest her for making a nuisance 9-1-1 call, she pretends she is having a heart attack. The firefighters on the scene each offer mouth-to-mouth resuscitation. She first says no to the Muslim woman and then the gay man. She points to Paul, proclaiming that she is not racist since he is African American. She then asks Paul if he is gay. He says no, much to her relief. He then tells her he is transgender. Having run out of minority groups to insult, she puts up her wrists to be handcuffed and says "Take me to jail" as everyone laughs.

While transphobic jokes can be used to disparage characters and perpetuate stereotypes, humor, such as gentle teasing, can be used to call out bad behavior without making the offending party feel defensive. For example, as Adam (*Degrassi*) and Missy are kissing, the cucumber Adam had put in his pants falls to the floor. Later, Missy suggests they get dinner and jokes, "Hold the pickles." Jake's (*Tales of the City*) younger nephew calls out "Aunty Jake! Aunty Margot!" when they arrive. The nephew's older brother corrects him, "It's *Uncle* Jake now." The nephew then overcorrects and shouts, "Uncle Jake! Uncle Margot!" Tess, Randall and Beth's daughter, is dating a nonbinary teen on *This Is Us*. Randall calls out Beth, who is mumbling to herself, "You are practicing Alex's gender pronouns right now, aren't you?" Beth responds, "Hell yeah, you know Tess is mean when you get those wrong." Beth's overbearing mother corrects her in a sarcastic tone, "Bethany, Alex is a teenager, not the gender police."

The following examples follow the incongruity theory of humor while easing the tension of coming out. TK and his boyfriend Carlos are taking Paul (*9-1-1: Lone Star*) out after work. Paul, worried about how others will react to the fact that he is transgender, says to Carlos, "I guess [TK] told you about me," to which Carlos answers, "That you're straight? I don't judge." Micah (*The L Word Generation Q*) takes Jose to a nice restaurant on their first date. They have the following exchange:

MICAH: I don't think I can make it all the way through dinner without telling you something first . . .
JOSE: I know. You're trans. I saw you on Grindr.
MICAH: . . . I have a gift card.
JOSE: I am so sorry.
MICAH: You hate the gift card?
JOSE: No, I feel so stupid for saying the thing I said.

In another case of relieving tension, Mafee is trying to get his intern Taylor (*Billions*) to take a full-time position with the firm, so he orders lunch for them. Taylor, seeing what Mafee has selected for them, asks him, "What makes you think I'm a vegan?" Mafee, not wanting to come across as stereotyping Taylor for being nonbinary, fumbles, "I don't know, everything? All of it? Fuck! You're not?" Taylor pauses, letting Mafee sweat, and finally lets him off the hook: "Of course, I'm a vegan." After Aaron (*The Fosters*) comes out to her, Callie says, "I have a friend who is transgender." Aaron counters, "Really? You are going to give me the 'I have a friend who is transgender' speech. You know we don't all know each other, right?" After a pause, Aaron admits he does know Cole. In all these cases, there is an element of misunderstanding rather than targeted disparagement of transgender individuals.

Transgender comedian Ian Harvie, who plays transmasculine characters Michael (*Mistresses*) and Dale (*Transparent*), shares some humorous comeback lines in his live one-hour stand-up comedy special "May the Best Cock Win." I include some jokes from the special to highlight the similarity to some of the dialogue in the shows discussed earlier. Harvie explains that when he gets questions such as "You were born a woman?" he retorts, "No, I was born a baby." When overhearing "Does that dude have a dick?" Harvie answers, "Yes, it's just not on me right now." He jokes about having a T-shirt made with "I have a vagina" and an arrow pointing down so he does not have to keep explaining his transition status. He references how "trans panic" disorder was used by defendants in a murder case as an excuse for killing a transgender woman. Harvie flips the script and jokes, "Trans panic is when you forget to take your testosterone and your period comes back."

Reality Television

Lovelock (2019), in describing the impact of reality television, explained, "[S]pecific conventions of reality TV—its intimacy and emotion, its investments in celebrity and the ideal of authenticity—have inextricably shaped the ways in which queer people have become visible in reality shows." Ehren (2015) argued that although reality television may help educate the public and normalize gender diversity, it relies heavily on exploitative tropes. While these types of shows were not included in my analysis, which focused on fictional portrayals, I found them helpful in understanding the overall landscape of transgender individuals on television. I broke down reality shows into the subgenres of talks shows, docu-shows, and competition shows.

Talk Shows

Studies of the talk show genre have documented the stigmatization of transgender identification in popular culture (Gamson, 2001; Riggs, 2014; Serano, 2007). One-time transgender guests are vulnerable in regard to the intensive question-and-answer format where the host controls the narrative. Many shows' goals are exploitative (e.g., *Jerry Springer*) or meant to focus on how enlightened the charismatic host is (e.g., Oprah Winfrey).

Jerry Springer is notorious for capitalizing on his audience's transphobia for ratings. He once claimed, "The best-of-the-best have always been transgender secrets. You never know what the reaction may be." In the May 20,

2010, episode entitled "Jerry's Big Gay Show," a cisgender man jumps out of his chair and begins to beat his transgender girlfriend on camera after she reveals her gender identity. Audience reactions range from laughing so hard they fall out of their seats to standing and cheering on the aggressor. Not to be outdone, Maury Povich ran several episodes exploiting transgender women, one entitled "Glamour Girls or Sexy Studs?" in 2009. He commented, "I can't think of another show that we have more fun with than the show we are going to do today. We invited 12 beauties to our stage today, and some of them were born female, some were born male, and it's up to me and you to decide who's who." Not only is he exploiting the contestants, he is treating others' gender identity as something to be ridiculed for entertainment.

Even Oprah Winfrey, who now produces transgender-friendly shows on her OWN cable channel, sensationalized gender identity during her talk show days. One example featured a 2010 interview with Dr. Christine McGinn, a transgender woman who performs gender-affirmation surgeries, and her cisgender wife, Lisa. In the opening of the show, Oprah announces to her audience:

> They are a lesbian couple raising four-month-old twins. While Lisa is the twins' biological mother, here's the bombshell. Here is the bombshell. Christine, the blonde mommy you just saw, actually fathered the twins. [Audience murmurs.] Whaaaaaa?! Yes, I said *fathered*. Well, you know, I've said many things and had multiple introductions on this show in 25 years. I've never said, been able to say, "Here is a mother who fathered her own children."

The repetition and vocal emphasis of "here is the bombshell" highlights the novelty, if not the exploitation, of the segment.

Talk shows featuring transgender men date back to Phil Donahue's interview with Jude Patton in 1976 and Geraldo Rivera's interview with Steve Dain in 1977. In 2007, Thomas Beatie, who underwent artificial insemination and became pregnant to carry a child for his infertile wife earning him news headlines like "World's First Pregnant Man," made the talk show rounds. Fifteen-year-old Ryan Cassata came out as transgender and appeared on a variety of shows as well in 2009. Cassata said in an interview that *The Tyra Banks Show* was a humiliating experience (cited in heinz, 2016). Banks asked him extremely personal questions about getting his period and wearing a binder. Dr. Drew Pinsky filling in on *Larry King Live* was more respectful to Cassata, using the "he" pronoun when speaking with Ryan. However, Pinsky used the "she" pronoun when referring to Ryan when speaking to Ryan's mother, who still referred to Ryan as her "daughter."

Buck Angel's talk show appearances contrast that of young Ryan Cassata. Angel is an adult film actor, sex educator, and motivational speaker. In his interview with Tyra Banks, she complimented him on his masculinity by saying it appears as if he would have "a big dick" (cited in Leighton-Dure, 2019), the implication being if he were a "real" man. Angel also made a guest appearance on Howard Stern's "What's My Secret" segment in 2006. In response to goading by Stern and his crew, Angel stripped from the waist down, showing his vagina, and rode the Sybian, which is a masturbation device usually reserved for Stern's female guests.

In perhaps a first for nonbinary individuals, Sally Jesse Raphael in 1989 interviewed an individual named Toby, who self-identified as "neuter" or a "genderless." Raphael asked, "Are you annoyed with me because I am this ignorant? 'Cause I think I am. Like a lot of people, I don't really understand a lot of this. Will you explain it? I have a million questions." She went on to comment, "It's almost like you got here from Mars. I'm beginning to feel like I'm in a sci-fi movie." Toby responded, "I feel that way too. The only difference is is that I am the stranger on your planet."

Docu-shows

These documentary-style television series allow more depth than interview shows, even if the transgender person still receives only one-time exposure. Documentary style shows such as *I Am Cait*, *I Am Jazz*, *Becoming Us*, *The TS Madison Experience*, *New Girls on the Block*, and *Real World Brooklyn* follow the lives of transgender female cast members. I focus on three reality shows that feature transgender men: *Queer Eye for the Straight Guy*, *Queer Eye*: *More than a Makeover*, and *Strut*.

Although the transgender men featured in the *Queer Eye* franchise appear in only one episode, the show revolves around them in their home environment—in contrast to other shows where the transgender person is a guest on a production set. *Queer Eye for the Straight Guy* (2006) featured Miles Goff, a 24-year-old transgender man, the first transgender person in the franchise's history. Limited by an hour-long episode, Booth (2011) criticized the show for giving the audience the impression that transitions are relatively unproblematic. Many jokes were made about one of the gay cisgender hosts Carson's manhood or lack thereof. For example, as Ted is introducing Miles, saying, "He was born a woman but identifies more as a man," the rest of the cast responds in unison, "Like Carson!" Carson later asks, "Where's the ladies' room?" When Miles's roommate says there are no ladies there, Carson responds, "Hello! I'm here!" Carson asks if he can do testosterone with Mile to give him bigger muscles. Through the teasing and Carson's antics, Miles holds his own. When Ted asks him if he can make

Carson butch, Miles responds, "I don't know if anybody can make Cason butch." The emphasis on Carson's lack of manhood as a gay man is in stark contrast to Miles's identification as a transgender man.

Throughout the episode, there was a particular emphasis on top surgery. Miles shares, "I can't wait to do the whole chop" while making a cutting motion across his chest. Carson kids, "You should do like a donor, like give your boobs to a flat-chested girl." Thom continues the joke theme when showing Miles and his transgender roommate their remodeled living room: "When you guys aren't thinking about removing your breasts, you can watch TV!" The *Queer Eye* (2018) reboot features a second transgender man, Skyler. In the episode, the cast makes significantly fewer jokes, although Tan teases Skyler about his style as being a "skater boy from 1995." Jonathan comments that he looks like a leprechaun, making fun of his red hair and beard. When Skyler comes out in a new outfit, the crew remark that they "classied the crazy."

Elements (2018), in a critique of the *Queer Eye* reboot, states that the franchise is still failing transgender men. The Skyler Jay episode (2018) opens with footage of Skyler's actual top surgery. Elements noted, "It makes it seem like all trans people need to be uncomfortable with their bodies or need to pursue medical transition in order to be valid in the eyes of cis folks." *Queer Eye* reboot cast members defended the episode, stating their mission was to help Skyler "become the man he was born to be." Karamo Brown thoughtfully added, "We support our sisters and brothers, but we don't know what they go through." The hosts at times make it more about themselves or act as stand-ins for an audience with little knowledge of the subject. Tan France, for example, repeatedly states that the experience was eye-opening and he was able to ask questions he's been dying to ask for years. In an interview following the episode, Skyler stated, "I don't blame Tan for his lack of knowledge. Instead, I very much thank him for his willingness to seek out that knowledge" (cited in Kaspar, 2018).

Despite all the joking (or perhaps because of it), *Queer Eye for the Straight Guy* received the GLAAD Media Award for Outstanding Reality Program in 2004 and 2005. While being criticized for the content of the Miles makeover, the show ended with a positive message for the viewers.

KYAN: Tolerance is okay, but acceptance is better.

JAI: You tolerate Mondays and jackhammers. People should be accepted.

THOM: Even when their views are different from yours.

TED: You may not understand everybody's culture or some of the personal decisions people make, but that's okay.

CARSON: Just remember, there is something we all want in common, peace and comfortable shoes.

Strut is a reality show about an all-transgender modeling agency, Slay. Laith Ashley is shown with his father sparring in a boxing ring (a demonstration of his masculinity). Ashley's mother is less accepting of his transition because of her religious beliefs. Near the end of the show's first and only season, she eventually acknowledges he is her "son." Ashley comments that they will transition together. In one episode, CeCe Asuncion, the director of scouting and development at Slay Model Management, steps in when the transgender female models are fawning over Ashley, the one transgender male cast member. Asuncion states, "I feel like I need to protect Laith from all the other models. It's seriously like dropping a steak in a cage full of lions. He is shy." On the surface, the aggressive behavior of the transgender women and the shyness of the transgender man might lead viewers to think that masculinity, expressed as aggression, and femininity, expressed as shyness, is inherent to the gender assigned at birth. However, if anyone has seen a bachelorette party recently or attended an all-male review, they would know that female audience behavior can be unsavory, to say the least (see Oppliger, 2008).

Competition Shows

Competition series allow for multiple appearances by transgender individuals—as long as they do not get voted off. Chaz Bono is credited for being the first transgender man on a competitive reality show when he appeared on *Dancing with the Stars* in 2011. Mocarski, Butler, Emmons, and Smallwood's (2013) analysis of his appearance notes that the men are often shirtless or at least have part of their shirt open; however, Bono is fully clothed in all six of his performances. The authors discuss his dances as choreographed in an "unsexed" manner," such that most of them end with him posing away from his partner. Mocarski and associates explain that he is "neutered" in the commentary and the judges' critiques. Carrie Ann Inaba, for example, referred to Bono as "cute" and "cuddly" and nicknamed him Chaziboy, which according to Mocarski et al. (2013), reinforces this "childlike construction" (p. 254). In addition, Judge Bruno Tonioli made references to his weight, likening him to a penguin and an Ewok.

Zeke Smith was a contestant on two seasons of the reality competition show *Survivor*, "Millennials vs. Gen X" in 2016 and "Game Changers" in 2017. In the second season, fellow contestant Jeff Varner outed Smith. Addressing Smith, Varner asked, "Why haven't you told everyone you are transgender?" The tribe backed up Smith by unanimously voting Varner off the show, saying the attack was personal. Smith responded, "I'm a changed, stronger man today than I was then. Varner, it's really not cool, but I'm fine." On behalf of the show, host Jeff Probst posted via Twitter, "Our hope is that this emotional and powerful conversation will bring awareness and understanding . . . and ultimately change" (cited in Allen, 2017). Varner then released a statement: "Let me be clear, outing someone is assault. It robs a strong, courageous person of their power and protection and opens them up to discrimination and danger" (cited in Allen, 2017).

In season 13 of *RuPaul's Drag Race*, Gottmik became the franchise's first-ever transgender man to compete, making the final four. The season premiere became the most-watched episode in the franchise's "herstory" (Ramos, 2021). RuPaul Charles had initially defended the show's policy of excluding transgender contestants, saying, "Drag loses its sense of danger and its sense of irony once it's not men doing it, because at its core it's a social statement and a big f-you to male-dominated culture" (cited in Framke, 2018). Charles later apologized for the comments. What is interesting is that it was not until deep into the series (the 10th episode) that Gottmik's transgender identity was discussed. In terms of the media's influence, Gottmik stated, "I really didn't see anyone like me ever on TV. And even when I did see the Chaz Bonos and trans guys on TV, I was just like that's too masculine. That is not me. I'm too feminine. If there was someone like me on TV when I was a kid, there would have been years shaved off my little journey" (cited in Charles, 2021).

Edu-tainment Factor

Something all genres have in common is their propensity to incorporate informative messages into the entertainment format. This treatment moves transgender character representation closer to Clark's final stage of respect. Siebler (2010) and Reed (2009) addressed how media shape culture and educate viewers regarding transqueer representations. In several interviews, writers and producers acknowledged making concerted efforts to enlighten audiences and treat transgender storylines with respect. Unlike films that exploit gender-diverse individuals for shock value or voyeuristic pleasure (see Phillips, 2006), many television shows are vehicles for introducing the challenges of fitting into a traditionally gendered, binary society (Oppliger & Medeiros, 2017). For example, producers created moments for the audience to learn about and empathize with the discrimination, frustration, and humiliation transgender people experience. These educational opportunities in scenes and plotlines are presented in a controlled environment where conversations can be practiced. *The Fosters* created an "alternative prom" to introduce other transgender and nonbinary characters. To help Ian (and the audience) understand variations of gender identity, Trevor (*Shameless*) introduces Ian to his LGBTQ alliance group, who go around the table and introduce themselves with a variety of gender labels and pronouns (e.g., demisexual, agender, and girlfag).

According to Michael Grassi (cited in Xtra, 2010), the goal for *Degrassi* writers was for the show to feel organic where queer characters are interacting in the hallways with other students and not like an after-school special or a public service announcement. When Adam came out to Clare and Eli, he gave them a long explanation of his transitional journey starting at around age four or five. In the next season, a new character Dave questions what he saw as Adam getting special privileges. Adam responds, "If you want me to go into the boringness about transgender brain development, I'd be glad to." Adam then compares discrimination he faces to that of "whites only" signs, as both are based on something individuals do not choose or cannot change. This is especially poignant since Dave is African American. Callie's (*The Fosters*) boyfriend AJ is also a common catalyst for introducing teachable moments on the show. For example, when Cole takes off his shirt at the beach and exposes his top surgery scars, AJ quietly asks Callie, "What happened to him?" AJ displays surprise and expresses his confusion about why Cole would harm himself on purpose. Callie rather condescendingly explains Cole's journey. She scolds AJ, "He's in a good place, finally, so don't go making him feel weird about it."

When JJ's (*Council of Dads*) grandmother cannot understand how her young grandson can "decide she's a boy," family friend Anthony steps in and explains, "I don't think he decided to be a boy. I think he just is a boy. That's how Scott [JJ's deceased father] explained it to me . . . We all should, you know, let JJ be JJ." In the scene, Anthony models his own process of understanding. At the beginning of the second season of *Chilling Adventures of Sabrina*, Harvey is supportive of Theo but is confused about his reveal. Harvey asks, "So, we just call her Theo now?" Roz responds, "No, no, we call *him* Theo. Theo might look like a girl, but he's not. He's a boy. And that's how he's always been. He's just . . . ready now. To live as himself. As Theo," which Harvey appears to accept. In *Shameless*, Ian is set up to ask Trevor very intrusive questions about his transition, particularly his breasts. Trevor responds that "they didn't belong on my body. If you had an extra thumb on your hand, wouldn't you want it gone?"

As for nonbinary characters, Cal teaches Jackson what it means for them to identify as nonbinary, a theme evident in the show's title, *Sex Education*. The explanation is much more detailed in this 2021 instance than the 2017 explanation on *Degrassi: Next Class*, where Yael is struggling with their nonbinary identity. In that case, a teacher informs Yael that the school supports are available for her and that questioning one's gender identity can come with depression and anxiety. Her friend Lola also guides them, relaying information she learned from internet vloggers.

New Amsterdam (2018) does a significantly more thorough job of explaining the transition of a transmasculine character than other medical dramas, which often focus on the surgical aspect. In the episode, transgender youth Shay's parents describe how depressed he had been and how after he socially transitioned, he started smiling and making friends. Even a spokesperson for *Law & Order: SVU* claimed the show "strives to start a conversation and educate viewers on topics that may not otherwise come to light on television" (cited in Ennis, 2015).

Talk shows hosts often say their goal is to educate. Singhal and Rogers (2003), on the other hand, described shows like *Jerry Springer* and *Survivor* as "entertainment-degradation" or "entertainment-perversion" rather than "entertainment-education." In contrast, Katie Couric apologized after she asked transgender model Carmen Carrera about her genitalia in a 2014 interview. After Carrera pushed back and refused to answer, Couric apologized. Couric refused to take out the segment, using it as a teachable moment. Lavern Cox reassured her, "It's only a mistake if you make it twice." Couric went on to produce the National Geographic special *Gender Revolution*, which explores evolving gender identity.

What was most interesting and educational about the reality show *Strut* was when Laith Ashley gets set up on a blind date. When he discloses his gender shortly after they meet, the date responds, "Amazing!" He appears comfortable with her questions until she asks him if he has a penis. He tenses up and tells her that is the one question cisgender people should not ask. "It's like me asking, 'Is your vagina really tight or really loose?'" After the date, Ashley explains, "It's inappropriate to ask anyone about their genitals." He reasons, "I had to realize that people just don't know. That's not an excuse but it's just the reality of the world."

Final Thoughts

Booth (2011) warned of sensationalizing transgender media representations for commercial gain. This is especially relevant because transgender characters are teaching audiences as they entertain. Producers of various genres focus on the novel aspect, which can easily cross over into exploitation. As these portrayals become more prevalent and familiar, more of the focus can be on the characters' personalities and less on their gender identification. It appears that the treatment is significantly different and has become more sensitive over time with more input from transgender writers, consultants, and actors. Although this was not a random sample, there is a clear pattern in the shows that feature ongoing transmasculine and gender-questioning characters. These representations, with the possible exception of Paul (*CSI*) in 2000, reveal a two-tier system where multi- and single-episode transgender characters are treated differently. In case after case, recurring characters are respected and normal, especially in newer series. They are portrayed as more than their gender identity.

4 How to Be Television Trans

Media rely on stereotypes to tell stories, especially when the topics deal with novel representations. At issue is the limited number of transmasculine characters, along with outdated tropes. I argue that the changes in the last decade have been progressively improving with the addition of more characters and the expansion of the kinds of stories that are told. The goal of this analysis is to explore how transgender and transmasculinity are defined in fictional television portrayals. This chapter includes a comparative analysis of characters of different ages, whose journeys are in various stages in the process of transitioning, and different time frames of the television series in which they appear. In this analysis, I note an emphasis on a range of themes from characters' identification (e.g., pronoun use, name changes) to physical expression (e.g. surgery, hormones) paralleling those listed by the American Psychiatric Association:

> People who are transgender may pursue multiple domains of gender affirmation, including social affirmation (e.g., changing one's name and pronouns), surgical affirmation (e.g., vaginoplasty, facial feminization surgery, breast augmentation, masculine chest reconstruction, etc.), medical affirmation (e.g., pubertal suppression or gender-affirming hormones), and/or legal affirmation (e.g., changing gender markers on one's government-issued documents).
>
> (Turban, 2020)

Social Affirmation

While it may appear to critics that labels reduce being transgender to superficial markers, naming and pronouns may be important first steps to developing an understanding of gender identity. Cavalcante (2018) noted that transgender terminology is central to articulating transgender experience. Nonbinary actor Blue del Barrio stated, "For many non-binary people,

DOI: 10.4324/9781003204404-4

myself included, finding the language to match what you feel can be very difficult. I didn't know the term existed until I was 21, but when I found it, my whole life suddenly made sense" (cited in Adams, 2020). As McInroy and Craig (2015) argued, shared vocabulary can create community. Cole on *The Fosters* explained that labels have power and that labeling himself as transgender was instrumental in getting him transferred to an LGBTQ group home where he could be his true self. The character added, "Sometimes labels can make us feel not so alone."

Television writers regularly stress terminology, naming, and pronouns, especially when dealing with novel concepts, which is still an unfamiliar subject to many audience members. Labels can clarify complex issues without having to invest in a great deal of explanation or backstory. *Grey's Anatomy* showrunner Krista Vernoff noted the lack of representation highlights the importance of naming characters' identities: "Most people have never seen a trans man. If you don't say 'trans man,' the people you most want to get this are going to miss it" (cited in Goldberg, 2018). Over time, writers appear to be changing with the culture and are adapting to more legitimate expressions of gender identity and more sensitive terminology. For example, the inclusion of tropes such as "born in the wrong body" are more likely to appear in early episodes while at the same time demonstrating increased acceptance of the transgender characters' preferred names and pronouns.

Language specific to gender identity allows characters to self-define rather than rely on other characters or audience members to correctly or incorrectly deduce their status from their physical appearance. *Shameless* writers made a point of introducing Ian to Trevor's LGBTQ group, which also informs viewers about a variety of labels and pronouns. Characters expressed their identities as "tri-racial, cisgender, girlfag. I identify as a pansexual, pronoun 'she'"; "gender-fluid, hetero-romantic, demisexual, and a redhead, pronoun 'he'"; "genderqueer, tax attorney"; and "I identify as Jennifer Anniston. Kidding. Agender, intersex, AFAB, pronoun 'they.'" These labels are comparable to the 58 gender-identification options Facebook began to offer users in 2014 beyond simply "male" or "female." When it came to gender markers in my sample, 32 characters discussed either or both name and pronoun changes, with only 12 not mentioning either.

Focus on Names and Pronouns

As a society, we also classify most names as male (e.g., Patrick) or female (e.g., Patricia). Part of the transition in television portrayals is the adoption of a chosen name that fits better with the characters' identity rather than the ones on their original birth certificates. Shows in this sample often used names that could be either gender, such as Sam, Max, Lex, Chris, Taylor,

Alex, Micah, Drew, Casey, Joey, Frankie, and Syd. While a vast majority of the characters had already adopted names that matched their gender identity when they first appeared, only five of the characters began the series with names given them at birth, switching to their preferred name during the run of the show (e.g., Max in *The L Word*, Sheldon in *Glee*, Theo in *Chilling Adventures of Sabrina*, Ben in *Good Girls*, Em in *Shrill*). Ben (*Good Girls*) recounts his stepmother saying his name over and over to prove she is accepting of his transition. Ben and his mother mock her, saying she is "so woke." Max (*The L Word*) crafts a message to his friends disclosing his transition. In addition to the statement, "Please only use the male pronoun when referring to me," Jenny recommends that he end with "Max, the transgender formerly known as Moira."

Names assigned at birth that are no longer used, often because of their implied gender, are referred to as deadnames. In an example of a name change to better reflect his true self, Michael (*Rise*) hesitantly writes "Margaret (Michael) Hallowell" on the theater tryouts signup sheet. Since the character now identifies as "Michael," the theater teacher scratches out the "Margaret" part, symbolizing acceptance of his social transition to transgender male. In *Degrassi*, one of the teachers calls out Adam's deadname while taking attendance. Seeing Adam's horrified response, the teacher corrects himself and calls out "Adam Torres." He apologizes, saying, "Wrong list." The use of deadnames can be hurtful to transgender individuals because it may bring up bad memories of their past struggles or put them in danger of transphobic attacks. The series *Work in Progress* addresses the use of deadnaming in a very touching manner. Abby picks up Chris' prescription bottle and sees his deadname (which is blurred so the audience can't see it). Chris has told Abby that she can ask him anything about his past except for his deadname. Fearing the repercussions, Abby hides the discovery from him, which is difficult for Abby because of her obsessive-compulsive disorder. When they go to get something to eat, Chris picks a café that happens to have the same name as his deadname. Abby suffers severe anxiety as she sees the name everywhere, on the cafe sign, the menu, and coffee cups. The pressure builds until she finally confesses. Chris tells Abby she is too much and walks away. She yells out his deadname. Chris is hurt and asks why she did it. Abby replies, "I wanted you to feel as broken as I am."

Gottmik (*RuPaul's Drag Race*) described his personal experience of naming:

> When someone calls me my deadname, my brain always just wants to ignore it so I don't have to talk to some random person I barely know about my life story for five minutes. But my friends have really helped

> me learn that it's not only important for them but for me to be correcting them and making sure I'm moving forward in this journey.
>
> (cited in Damshenas, 2021)

Ian Harvie incorporates his mother's continued use of his deadname in his stand-up comedy special. He jokes about her saying it out loud in a store to get his attention. The other shoppers were shocked when he answered to the name "Janet," especially since he presents as very masculine (i.e., facial hair).

As with other languages, English pronouns are gendered in the third-person singular. Changing pronouns or using the plural "they/them" for a nonbinary individual is proving to be a major stumbling block for some nontransgender individuals. Focusing on pronouns may appear superficial, but from a communication perspective, it has substantial meaning for defining one's sense of self. Booth (2015) argued, "While the inconsistent use of pronouns may appear to be an insignificant matter of etiquette, it indicates a foundational lack of understanding about transgender people that can lead not only to poor treatment interpersonally, but also to the passage of laws affecting how transgender people are able to live in the world" (p. 123). According to a Trevor Project survey in 2020, transgender and nonbinary youth were half as likely to attempt suicide if their pronouns were respected (Paley, 2020).

Television show writers can quickly establish characters' gender identity with pronoun dialogue. For example, the nonbinary character Riley (*The Red Line*) discloses their gender identity immediately in their first scene. They tell their best friend that it took all summer, but "Mom and Dad are solid with pronouns." They add their brother Jacob "acts like he's never used 'they' in his life." Pronoun selection can also be part of the discovery process. Lola (*Degrassi: Next Class*) discusses selecting a pronoun with Yael, who is exploring a nonbinary identity. Lola informs Yael, "Most people like you use different pronouns like 'ze' instead of 'he' or 'she.'" When Yael selects the pronouns "they/them," their boyfriend Hunter thinks it is ridiculous. He argues, "'They' is plural. Yael's not two people." His friend Baaz responds, "She . . . I mean, they seem happy, so does it matter what we call . . . them?" Sam (*Glee*) is a bit overzealous with the pronouns in response to Coach Beiste's transitions. "I have this list of all these pronouns, I mean just tell me which one and I'll enforce it. There's 'he,' there's 'shu-hee,' there's 'it, 'zee,' 'zeem.'"

The *One Day at a Time* episode "To Zir, With Love" gives the audience a crash course in pronoun use such as "they/them" and "ze/zir." Elena is organizing a protest and instructs them, "Okay, everybody! When we get there, she takes her team to the stairs, ze takes zir team to the parking lot, and they take their team to the corner. He, she, they, and ze will all meet up at the fair-trade coffee shop between the two Starbucks." Gottmik represents a novel case since Gottmik is the name of Kade Gottlieb's drag persona, whereas Kade identifies as a transgender man outside of drag. On the *Drag Race* aftershow *Whatcha Packing*, host Michelle Visage (2020) interviewed Gottmik about her experience on *RuPaul's Drag Race*, where the contestants are referred to as "she."

VISAGE: You are a trans man, so I kept not knowing what pronouns to use and did not want to misgender. But there's a conflict here because you are a man, but when you are in drag, you're a she. So, not to offend, I kept saying, "Gottmik, Gottmik," and then finally, they were like, "Michelle, you can calm down, she's okay about using the pronoun 'she' when she's in drag." Am I safe to say that?

GOTTMIK: Yes, a thousand percent. I don't know that many people that feel like me because I am transmasculine, super hard "he" out of drag, but I feel like if I was the only drag queen not getting called "she," I would be reverse clocking myself in a way.

There are three characters who present challenges in terms of standard labeling and pronouns, in that there is no mention of the characters expressing their preferred pronouns, only references made by others. Roscoe (*House of Lies*) explains to his father, who is confused about the gender status of Roscoe's friend Lex, that Lex was born a girl but is a "boi" or a "grrl." Roscoe uses the "he/him" pronouns for Lex yet refers to Lex as his "girlfriend." Frankie (*Better Things*) and Dolly (*Gypsy*) also do not fit neatly into categories. There is no mention of changing names or pronouns. Both characters' families continue to use "she/her" pronouns. In an interview, *Better Things* creator Pamela Adlon said she has purposely avoided giving Frankie any definitive labels. "I've always felt on both sides of the line in terms of the way I feel about myself" (cited in Malcon, 2020).

Sexual Orientation

People often conflate sexual orientation with gender identity. Gender specialist Diane Ehrensaft, Ph.D. (2016) explained, "Children who mix up gender in their dress, in their play, and in their self-declaration as 'boy,' 'girl,' or 'other' are telling us information about their gender, not their sexuality." According to GLAAD (n.d.), gender identity is "your own, internal, personal sense of being a man or a woman (or as someone outside of that gender binary)." Sexual orientation describes a person's enduring physical, romantic, and/or emotional attraction to another person (e.g., straight, gay, lesbian, bisexual). This difference is highlighted in a scene in *Glee* where Kurt, a gay cisgender male character, tries to talk Unique, a transfeminine character (who still presents as male at times), out of performing in a dress and heels for fear she will be ridiculed. Kurt tries to empathize with the situation by pointing out he has worn some flamboyant outfits, although he has never dressed up as a woman. Unique responds, "That's because you identify yourself as a man. I thought you, of all people, would understand."

Ellis (2020) argued that some producers do not appear to have put much thought into acknowledging that transgender people have a sexual orientation like their cisgender counterparts. In contrast, 34 out of the 44 characters in my sample acknowledged or self-label their sexual orientation. Twenty characters expressed or demonstrated their attraction to cisgender women, ten to cisgender men, three to both cisgender women and cisgender men, and one to a nonbinary AFAB character. Of the 11 nonbinary characters, six dated or showed interest in ciswomen, three to cisgender men, and two dated both cisgender women and cisgender men. Of the 23 transgender men in the sample who expressed romantic interests, 13 dated, kissed, married, or were divorced from cisgender women; six dated cisgender men only; three dated both cisgender men and cisgender women; and one transgender man dated a nonbinary character. Three characters who were in what they self-identify as lesbian relationships before their transitions to transgender men subsequently had sexual relationships with cisgender men.

Romantic relationships and attractions call attention to sexual orientation labels. The first three letters of LGBTQ signify sexual orientation, which signifies a binary perspective on gender. I refrained from labeling characters who did not disclose their sexual orientation since their apparent attraction to specific characters does not exclude attraction to other characters with differing gender identities. Two characters in the sample introduced the label "queer" (the Q in LGBTQ) to describe their relationships. For example, Jake (*Tales of the City*), a transgender man, tells his partner Margot, a cisgender woman who identifies as a lesbian, that "they are queer now" after his transition. Cal (*Sex Education*) explains to Jackson that if they are going to be in a relationship, Jackson, a cisgender boy, will be queer because Cal identifies as nonbinary. If he continues to identify as heterosexual, it signifies to Cal that he sees them as a girl, which they are not. Another example of sexual orientation labels with nonbinary identified individuals or nonbinary partners is included in the series *One Day at a Time*. Cisfemale Elena comes out to her family as a lesbian early in the series. After initially referring to her nonbinary partner as her "girlfriend," the writers of the show seemed to have adjusted their perspective. In a later episode, they have the couple discuss choosing a different term instead of "girlfriend" for Syd. However, Elena continues to identify as a lesbian and a "girl who likes girls." *Degrassi: Next Class* explores the sexuality of a nonbinary character and their relationship with their boyfriend as they transition. Yael, who is struggling with their gender identity, kisses Lola to see if they are a lesbian. A group of students contemplates back and forth, questioning whether Yael is now bi, poly, or perhaps pan after they come out as nonbinary. As another alternative to standard labels, Marty (*House of Lies*) asks Roscoe about dating Lex, whose gender identity trends toward transmasculine: "So what does that make you?" Roscoe simply responds, "Roscoe?"

Defining Masculinity

In the series *Degrassi*: *Next Generation*, the cismasculine character Dave asks the transmasculine character Adam, "So, the question here is what makes you a guy exactly?" Adam quips back, "No, the question is what makes you a guy?" Merriam Webster's Dictionary (2021b) defines masculine as "having qualities appropriate to or usually associated with a man." According to Nick Adams of GLAAD, "If a show's going to tell a story about kids whose gender expression is something other than typically masculine or feminine, it's important that they know the difference between gender expression and gender identity" (cited in Friedland, 2018). Stryker (2017) offered definitions for various terms: "gendered appearance of the body" as in taking hormones; "gender expression," how we perform our sense of self or "gender identity"; and "gender presentation," making gender diversity visible. The process of transitioning can range in scope, from changing how one dresses to legally changing one's name to medical procedures, such as hormone therapy or reassignment surgery (Turban, 2020). Television plot points tend to incorporate these factors. The following is an analysis of the various external and internal expressions of masculinity.

Surgical

Noble (2004) argued that the difficulty of forming and surgically attaching a penis impedes transgender men from "leaving the 'trans' behind and being just 'men.'" Booth (2015) proposed that even though most transgender men do not get phalloplasty (taking tissues from the forearm to construct a penis) because of the cost and scarring, many television viewers "insist upon genital surgery as a validation of gendered identity." Booth framed surgery as a rite of passage from one gender identity to another. While none of the characters in my sample has apparently had bottom surgery, there were several mentions of "top surgery" (i.e., masculinizing chest surgery). In response to Ian's (*Shameless*) inquiry about Trevor's breasts, Trevor explains, "Yeah, I got them the fuck chopped off. Best day of my life. They didn't belong on my body." Transmasculine actors cast in the roles of trans men allow audiences to see top surgery scars, one sign of how "masculinity" is expressed. On *The Fosters*, Tom Phelan, who plays Cole, had his surgery during the run of the series and takes off his shirt during a beach scene and exposes his scars. In another episode, Callie is sketching a shirtless Aaron. When she leaves off his scars, he tells her to add them to the portrait because he finally loves his body and needs to tell his story. On the reality show *Queer Eye* (2018), Skyler shares that it was necessary for him to have chest masculinization surgery to feel like a man. Skyler takes his shirt off on the dance floor, in addition to showing video of his surgery at the beginning of the episode. The character Max (*The L Word*), on the other hand, reveals that he decides not to go through with the surgery he scheduled. Theo (*Chilling Adventures of Sabrina*) likewise states that he does not have to change his body to feel like a boy. Booth (2015) noted that how one identifies and how one desires to live is separate from one's current or future surgical status, which these last two examples illustrate.

As an alternative to surgically adding a penis, television series include other types of phallic references. To make Adam (*Degrassi*) appear more masculine, his brother Drew gives Adam his leather jacket and sprays him with body spray. He tells Adam that he should put a cucumber in his pants for his date with Missy in case she gets "grabby." When Ian asks if Trevor has a penis, Trevor (*Shameless*) tells Ian he is "packing" and gives a detailed explanation of his dildo collection. *Transparent* spends significant screen time showing Dale shopping for and attempting to use a dildo in a bathroom sex scene. Much of the dialogue in that episode matches material in Harvie's stand-up act and thus his personal experience. Even though he does not have an attached penis, he tells the audience he can go out and buy his girlfriend exactly what she wants, hence the title of his stand-up show "May the Best Cock Win." He further jokes that ever since he has been on testosterone, he walks down the street thinking, "I would put my dick in that . . . I'm so gross now!" Somewhat related, standing urination is promoted as a sign of masculinity. Max on *The L Word* tells Jenny that he has peed standing up since he was little. Max tells her it makes him feel like a real guy. He has a device called Pissin Passin' Packer. Fitz and Owen harass Adam (*Degrassi*) in the boys' restroom, taunting him "whip it out." In the next season, Adam pulls out a stand-to-pee device he purchased online.

Hormone Therapy

Testosterone is used as an alternative or complement to surgery in media representations. Adam (*Degrassi*) asks his mother about starting testosterone. He envies his cismasculine friend Dallas who has upper body muscles, facial hair, and a deep voice. Adam is especially jealous of his girlfriend's new friend after seeing pictures of his bare muscular chest. Paul's (*9-1-1: Lone Star*) mother says to him, "Look at you! Is this my son or Vin Diesel? Naomi, doesn't your brother look strong? Ooh, feel these biceps." It is evident that both the character Paul and Brian Michael Smith, the transgender man who plays Paul, take testosterone. *Queer Eye* (2006) makeover subject Miles explains that he went on testosterone for what he considers selfish reasons. "I was always correcting people about my pronoun, and that automatically put me in the position of having to educate them. I know that this depresses me, to not pass as a guy and to have to constantly be defending my maleness."

Villarreal (2020) outlined problematic stereotypes of Max on *The L Word* as he transitions to male. "The show made Max's transition an oversimplified affair with Max taking a testosterone shot in one episode and scheduling transitional surgery barely two episodes later. Over a two-week period, he grows a mustache and beard which is pretty much impossible." The series also emphasizes the stereotypical effects of hormone use. Shortly after Jenny gives Max his first dose of testosterone, Max says he is feeling edgy and horny. In his support group, the transgender men talk about how they can't cry anymore because of the hormones. Max begins to experience roid rage. He scares Jenny when he yells at her. He later goes into a jealous rage when Jenny dances with someone else, grabbing her arm. When Star (*David Makes Man*) tosses David a bottle of water, he throws it so hard that David is unable to catch it. Fammie tells Star, "You need to take less T, sir. All aggressive for no reason." Coach Beiste (*Glee*) explodes when confronted about skipping out on practice. In contrast to these portrayals, Stanford neuroscientist Robert Sapolsky dispelled the myth that testosterone causes aggression. Instead, he explained that testosterone "causes 'status-seeking' behavior that our culture rewards aggression with status" (cited in heinz, 2016). On the positive side, shows warn of the dangers of self-medicating. Because he is a minor and in the foster care system, Cole (*The Fosters*) does not have access to doctor-prescribed hormone therapy. After illegally acquiring street hormones, he is hospitalized for a bad reaction to the drugs.

Visible Gender Cues

Gender ascriptions are often based on distinguishable physical characteristics. For example, body hair is a sign of masculinity and an indicator of puberty, a time when sex differences become more defined. Margot sketches a picture of Jake (*Tales of the City*) but goes back and erases his facial hair. Jakes becomes upset when he sees the altered sketch. Margot confesses, "I know I'm not allowed to, but I miss her." Kyan says to Miles on *Queer*

Eye for the Straight Guy (2006), "Your beard is kind of like your trophy. You've earned it." Skyler (*Queer Eye*, 2018) describes his beard as the first thing that made him "visually feel like a man." Jonathan explains how the length of Skyler's beard, instead of making him manlier, makes his jawline appear more feminine. Jonathan leaves a shadow of facial hair so Skyler can still feel masculine. In terms of hair on other parts of the body, Kyan compliments Miles on the underarm hair he has developed since he has been on testosterone. In contrast, nonbinary character Yael's (*Degrassi: Next Class*) armpit hair was photoshopped out of their yearbook photo. Yael pushes back, saying they are not embarrassed about their armpit hair, and they refuse to shave their legs, noting that the boys don't shave there. Yael's boyfriend Hunter confronts Yael for acting differently and not shaving. Sam becomes suspicious of Coach Beiste's (*Glee*) extra leg hair, not knowing he has begun hormone treatment.

For Theo's character in *Chilling Adventures of Sabrina*, his father taking him to get a haircut marks his acceptance of Theo's transition. Jean at first denies her nine-year-old daughter Dolly's (*Gypsy*) request to get her hair cut. She tells Dolly that she has beautiful hair. Dolly does not take it as a compliment, pointing out that no one thinks the action figure G.I. Joe has beautiful hair. Dolly ends up cutting her own hair, explaining to her mother, "I wanted to look like me." There is also strong symbolism of femininity in a hair clip. Adam (*Degrassi*) wears a hair clip to symbolize his pre-transition self. He uses it to self-harm, heating it with a lighter and repeatedly burning his arm. Sam, on the series *The Riches*, uses the same symbolism to demonstrate gender expression by having him put a hair clip in his hair when expressing his feminine identity.

Clothing is another substantial form of gender expression. Ben's father is concerned when a pre-transition Ben (*Good Girls*) is getting bullied at school for wearing bowties. His mother downplays it and attributes it to Ben figuring out who he is. Adam's (*Degrassi*) mother insists they go shopping to get something feminine to wear for Adam's grandmother, who is not aware of Adam's transition. Adam's friends stage a ceremonial bonfire to burn his "girl" clothes. As a sign of accepting Adam's new gender identity, his family joins them. On the reality makeover show *Queer Eye* (2006), Miles explained that it is difficult to find men's clothing that fits because of his small stature. He discloses that it is awkward when he must shop in the little boys' section for something that will fit. In 2018 Skyler has similar issues. One of the *Queer Eye* hosts introduces him to a friend who has a company that tailors suits for transgender men to reduce and straighten the hips.

In some cases, clothing is more than just gender expression, as it can affect one's internal gender identity. In *Degrassi: Next Class*, Yael discloses, "I don't feel like a girl or what everyone thinks is a girl." Lola gives them a makeover, dressing Yael in a vest with a white T-shirt and slouchy jeans. Yael looks at themself in the mirror, sighs, and starts to cry. Lola worries that she did something wrong. Yael tells her, "No, no. You did it exactly right." As a nonbinary student, Cal (*Sex Education*) rejects the school's gender-specific uniform. They not only feel uncomfortable wearing the girls' uniform (i.e., skirt), they wear an oversized boys' uniform that is not so form-fitting.

By adopting the look of traditionally cisgender individuals, one is thought to "pass" for that gender, an expression often used in cross-dressing movies. heinz (2016) defined passing as "external recognition and validation of one's masculine identification and notions of completeness as in one's internal validation of one's masculine identification" (p. 196). Davidmann (2010) criticized the term passing for implying that a transgender individual is committing an "act of secrecy and dishonesty" and "playing a part no one has a right to play" (p. 191). It was rare to hear the expression "passing" in the sample, especially in more recent episodes. In 2012, Clare congratulated Adam (*Degrassi*) for passing as a gay guy. This concept of passing is not always portrayed as a compliment. Trevor (*Shameless*) deals with multiple references by the Gallagher family to his appearance, although the term "passing" is not used explicitly:

IAN: Sorry, it's just that . . . you look so much like a dude.
TREVOR: That's cool since I am a dude.
LIP (Ian's brother): Wow. I mean, you would have never known. I mean, you look real.
TREVOR: You look real, too.
MONICA (Ian's mother): You're trans? I couldn't tell.
TREVOR: Thanks [sarcastically].

Trevor's responses to the Gallaghers, a "scrappy, feisty, fiercely loyal Chicago family [who] makes no apologies" (IMDB, n.d.), demonstrate incredible patience and a sense of humor.

Macho Talk/Hypermasculine Behavior

Besides physical traits, masculinity is expressed through macho talk and hypermasculine behavior. As expressions of masculinity on *The L Word*, Max is shown in a jumpsuit and bandana around his head, working on a car. In other scenes, he is lying on a bench lifting weights or working the grill at a cookout. Masculinity also means treating phallus and penis size as a measurement of manhood. Taylor (*Billions*) explained why they stopped playing poker online, "That whole my dick is bigger than your dick thing, it just wasn't for me. I'm already stewarding a firm. A bigger one, not that size matters."

Fighting, in particular, is presented as a sign of masculinity. When April's boyfriend Mark punches Michael (*Mistresses*) for kissing April, Michael is actually glad, explaining it was an authentic moment for him as a man. Miles (*Queer Eye*) kills a fly in his bathroom with his hand, to which Carson exclaims, "That was so butch." Miles jokingly replies, "I'm a manly man now." Other characters appear to misunderstand the transmasculine characters' desire to fight or fail to take them seriously when they do fight. To protect Sasha, Michael (*Rise*) grabs Sasha's boyfriend by the shirt and pushes him. Sasha responds, "You were trying to be a guy doing something you think some guy would do. I don't even know who you are anymore." After a rival band group tries to kick them out of their band rehearsal space, Theo (*Chilling Adventures of Sabrina*) comes at their leader: "How about I beat your sad ass?" Harvey pulls him back. Harvey later recounts the incident to Sabrina as they laugh, obviously not taking Theo seriously. When Adam (*Degrassi*) wants to join Fitz's fight club, Fitz will only allow Adam to fight girls. Adam gets upset and punches Fitz to demonstrate his masculinity. In another scene, Adam punches a rival band member. Guest judge Chaz Bono tells Adam is it is not okay to fight, even if the other guy made fun of Adam for being transgender.

Masculinity can also be expressed through "guy talk" or gendered senses of humor. As Adam (*Degrassi*) is establishing himself with boys at his new school, he feels the need to exert hypermasculinity. Eli describes how he was able to get an appointment at a body shop to get a taillight fixed. When Sav comments "I can't believe you got it in there," Adam comes back with "Yeah, that's what my ex-girlfriend said." Sav and Eli look puzzled. Eli calls him gross, while Sav simply ignores him. At another point in the conversation, Adam shouts, "Boo-yah!" Sav responds, "Dude, 'Boo-yah?'" Eli asks, "Who are you?" Adam is attempting to fit in with the guys since he is not out yet; however, Sav and Eli are confused by his over-the-top behavior. Eli is unfazed by Adam's later transgender disclosure. He asks if that means he can "rip one" in front of Adam. Adam replies, "Eli, I'd be insulted if you didn't." Yael (*Degrassi: Next Class*), who is questioning their gender, explains, "Me finding farts gross literally has nothing to do with my genitals and everything to do with the fact that they're disgusting."

Transmasculine characters are shown putting down cisgender boys in order to feel masculine. Adam is upset that Eli bailed on guys' night. When Fitz begins disparaging Eli, "Probably blinded himself with too much 'guy-liner,'" Adam joins in: "Yeah, probably listened to emo and got all emotional." Adam makes fun of Eli's feminine attributes, likely to elevate his own masculinity. Lex (*House of Lies*) acts in a similar way. When he and Roscoe are wrestling on the floor, Lex asks, "Is that all you got, little man? Come on, pretty boy." Lex is rude to Roscoe's friend, Coltrane, calling him "jazz hands." Lex is getting overly physical on the basketball court and chest-bumping others. Another friend, Ethan, challenges him, "Hey, Lex. Overcompensate much?' Lex responds by calling him a "pussy." Lex grabs Coltrane and kisses him. When Roscoe refuses to kiss Coltrane as well, Lex calls Roscoe a "faggot."

Negotiating Masculinity in Binary Portrayals

Sometimes, the representation of gender is defined by what it is not. Traditionally gender has been treated not on a continuum but as mutually exclusive concepts where femininity and masculinity are binary. This way of thinking may thus preclude others from fully perceiving transgender men as men. For example, there are clear gender distinctions at Jake's (*Tales of the City*) parents' house. His mom tells him to go watch the soccer game with his dad instead of helping her in the kitchen: "Doing dishes isn't for you anymore." His father and his Uncle Mando tease Jake's brother-in-law Stewart about his allergies, accusing him of crying. Mando tells Jake, "Hey, Dr. Rodriguez. Can you help Stewart grow a pair?" His dad jokes, "Don't be stupid. You can't grow a pair." There is also clearly a gender reference since Mondo calls him "Doctor," although Jake is in nursing school. When Jake begins to lose patience with their joking, Mando tells him to lighten up and have a beer unless he wants a wine cooler. He insists if Jake is going to hang out with the boys, he has to be able to "take some shit" and not be so sensitive. In a similar vein, Sue offers Coach Beiste (*Glee*) a shoulder to cry on after his transition, "metaphorically of course because you are a man now and real men don't cry."

While transitioning for some characters means full-on manliness, other characters are caught between their current masculinity and their former femininity. For example, Alice tells Max (*The L Word*) that he is going to be a very caring father because he knows what it is like to be both sexes. On *The L Word* reboot *Generation Q*, Jose tells Micah he has never been able to talk with someone like this before. Micah responds, "Well, I used to be a lesbian before." Ali (*Transparent*) calls Dale "gender enlightened" because he has basically experienced the world as two genders. Dale jokes, "I'm like a double agent." In some situations, cisgender women mistakenly think the men are cisgender, yet they sense a difference. Brooke notes that Max (*The L Word*) really understands women. Josie (*9-1-1: Lone Star*) tells Paul, "You know you're not like most of the guys around here. You're thoughtful, charming, sexy as hell. You are literally the man of my dreams." Yet she cannot get past his being transgender. April (*Mistresses*) is initially attracted to Michael. After he comes out, April's friend suggests she bonded with Michael on some deeper female level. April agrees that makes sense, like "a sisterhood thing." When deciding whether to continue her relationship with Bill (*Two and a Half Men*), Evelyn figures, "Well, he certainly understands women. He's gorgeous, he can afford beachfront property, and he's got a trunk full of fabulous shoes that fit me perfectly . . . Don't wait up. Mommy's got a date." These examples lead to questions such as the following: Are transgender men the best men because they have some innate ability to understand women? Are transmasculine characters seen as superior to cisgender males when it comes to admirable qualities? To what degree is gender a matter of being socialized as female rather than a biological effect?

Transition Narratives

heinz (2016) explained traditional transmasculine narratives in the following stages: emergence of trans consciousness, severe distress, treatment of the condition, and resolution of the distress and "integration into normative society" (p. 104). The severe distress aspect is likely presented in two forms: others' judgments and one's own perception that they need to be "fixed." The "wrong body" trope, according to Halberstam (1998), describes an error of nature "whereby gender identity and biological sex are not only discontinuous but catastrophically at odds." heinz (2016) added, "If one is trapped in the 'wrong' body, then one's condition needs to be 'righted'" (p. 89), which then leads to the third stage of altering the body through surgery and hormones. This "wrong body" trope is mainly found in older series, such as *The L Word*, *Degrassi*, and *The Fosters*. It no longer appears after 2015. Instead of "wrong body," Ian Harvie jokes in his comedy special, "I just feel like this was the right body. I just made some modifications to it."

Siebler (2012) argued that dominant narrative equates "trans" with "transitioning." In my sample, 30 out of 44 characters appeared at a stage of their transition where they were already comfortable with their identities. Only nine characters came out during their run in the series, while five who were out continued to struggle. What emerged from my analysis was that the timing in the series was a factor, more so than the age of the character.

The age of the characters has been a factor in past representations. Studies have shown that transgender characters are disproportionately older adults, with few representations of transgender youth (see Capuzza & Spencer, 2017; McInroy & Craig, 2015). This trend was not evident in my sample. Twenty-five characters were college-age or younger (four preteen, 18 teenagers, and three college-age) versus 19 older characters (eight were in their mid to late 20s; 11 were in their 30s or 40s). Many of the younger characters were still dependent on their parents emotionally and financially, which greatly affected their options. There are also more health considerations when it comes to gender confirmation surgeries, hormone treatments, and puberty blockers for adolescents.

I predicted a negative correlation between the age of the characters and their comfort level with their gender identity, but no distinct pattern emerged. For example, I compared the youngest character, six-year-old JJ (*Council of Dads*), with the oldest character, Coach Beiste (Glee), who is in his late 40s. JJ, who had fully transitioned socially, is portrayed as wise beyond his years. He tells his grandmother, who repeatedly misgenders him, that he is not mad at her and that it can take people from her generation a while to understand. He also maturely expresses his wish that transphobic parents "would just get their act together." It is not until the sixth season of *Glee* that Coach Beiste transitions after being on the show since season two. The character is presented as a female football coach for the first 40 episodes. After his coming out, he explains his confusion growing up, thinking he was just a tomboy. He started coaching football and wrestled hogs to express what he was feeling inside. After his transition on-screen (he was played by cisgender actor Dot-Marie Jones), he appeared in seven episodes before the show ended.

There has been a clear progression in regard to the representation of transgender characters over time. The earliest character in my sample was Paul Millander, who appeared in a three-episode arc of *CSI: Crime Scene Investigation* in 2000–2001. I hesitated to include him in my sample because his gender identity was not revealed until the third episode; however, his gender identity was given significantly more screen time than other crime procedural show transgender characters. His story was told through hazy flashbacks. According to the script, he suffered from "endocrinic ambiguity" at birth; therefore, his parents were told they could decide whether to raise him as a boy or a girl. His mother's rejection following his gender reassignment surgery contributed to his becoming a serial killer, a common trope on crime dramas.

In 2006, a pre-transition Max joined the cast of *The L Word.* He initially presents as a lesbian in the series before coming out as transgender. He begins to take street testosterone, and shortly after, he starts having aggressive episodes. The lesbian community questions his desire to transition to a man, asking, "Why he can't just be butch?" Max responds that he wants to "feel whole" and for the "outside to match the inside." He later becomes pregnant and is denied an abortion because he is too far along in the pregnancy. He describes the process: "All these things are happening to my body, and they totally go against how I feel about myself." The series ends before he gives birth. While Reed (2009) credited the story arc as educational, other critics disparaged the portrayal stating, "*L Word* is making it look as if the natural progression for butch women is to eventually become transgender" (Edwards, 2010, p. 168). Similar criticism was leveled at *Glee* (2015) for not maintaining Coach Beiste's character as a masculine-presenting female football coach. Another early character (2010) in *Degrassi*, Adam, is played by a cisgender actor and includes many "wrong body" tropes. The expression appears to disappear after 2015. The last year that a cisgender actor played a transgender character in this sample was 2017.

Questioning and Gender-Fluid Characters

Two of the characters in the sample, Dolly (*Gypsy*) and Frankie (*Better Things*), defy labels. As mentioned earlier, they retain "she/her" pronouns while presenting more masculine in hair and dress. In *Gypsy*, nine-year-old Dolly is not explicit in her masculine identity other than insisting she is not a girl. Dressed in flannel shirts, ball caps, ties, and cardigan sweaters, Dolly obsesses about *Star Wars* and playing a Jedi. In contrast to her friend Sadie's princesses and *Frozen*-themed birthday party, Dolly's party has no theme, with anything pink avoided "like the plague." Other than shorter hair, there is little change in her character's gender presentation over the course of the show's one and only season. She appears comfortable with who she is. It is her mother, Jean, who appears to adapt and change over the course of the series. Although she insists that she is allowing Dolly to express herself, she resists Dolly cutting her hair. In the end, Jean cuts Dolly's hair as short as she wants, a symbol of Jean's acceptance.

At the end of the first season of *Better Things*, Sam is called to the principal's office because her daughter Frankie, who is approximately 12 years old, was caught using the boys' restroom. Frankie insists that she is not a boy and does not need a unisex bathroom. She explains, "I know that is what people are saying. Like 'oh Frankie, oh obviously she is identifying as a boy, blah, blah, blah.'" Frankie appears comfortable in her short hair and masculine dress (e.g., pants, button-down shirts, and vests). It is her mother and her older sister Max who appear concerned. After the bathroom incident, Max tells Sam, "Mom, come on. Frankie's a boy." Sam simply replies, "Shit." There is no further mention of Frankie's gender identity until season four. Sam finds Frankie with a boy in her room. Sam, apparently conflating gender identity with sexual preference, confronts Max, "I thought you said Frankie was a boy." To confuse matters further, Max denies she never said that.

In contrast to Dolly and Frankie's comfort level, Lex (*House of Lies*) struggles with his public and private identification. He dresses in skirts at home, where his family still refers to him by his female name. With Roscoe, his gender-fluid boyfriend, he is dominant, pressuring Roscoe to hurry up and change, or he will leave without him. He is aggressive with other boys on the basketball court and eventually pushes Roscoe away with his hypermasculine behavior.

Diverse Gender Identification Struggles

Early in their appearance on *Degrassi: Next Class*, Yael hints at gender diversity. They begin complaining about pain from their breasts in gym class and progress to distinguishing themself from female-presenting classmates who care about makeup and nail polish. With the help of their cisgender friend Lola, Yael slowly realizes that they might not identify as female but rather as something in-between. After Lola gives them a makeover, Yael starts to cry and exclaims that Lola did it "exactly right." Yael adopts the "they/them" pronouns and declares that they are not going back. Bishop in *Deputy* also struggles with coming to terms with being nonbinary. After a serious car accident, they reassess their gender identity: "Until recently, I didn't have a word for what I felt like on the inside. I let people assume. I didn't want to make anyone else feel uncomfortable, but that just made me feel worse. You know, I hate labels, and here I am trying to give myself one." After confiding in their doctor, a relieved Bishop states, "I had no idea how badly I needed to say that to someone." Bishop, who is going by just their last name anyway, lets the others know of their preferred pronouns. They lose their girlfriend over the transition but gain another, more accepting one before the end of the series.

At the beginning of season two of *Good Trouble*, Joey tells their girlfriend, Alice, they are thinking of changing their pronouns to "they/them." They start wearing a binder and explain to Alice that they are not comfortable with their chest. Alice, noticing that Joey is presenting more masculine, deals with her discomfort by talking about Joey's transition in her standup comedy act, which offends Joey. They break up with Alice, telling her, "You don't have to get it. I don't expect someone who's comfortable in their gender identity to get it, but you do have to get me."

The Reveal

There is agency in deciding when, how, and whose story to tell. According to Booth (2015), "For transgender individuals, the communication of identity often begins with personal narrative, as delivered to friends and loved ones." The reveal is a narrative technique in literature and film and is "a moment in a trans person's life when the trans person is subjected to the pressures of a pervasive gender/sex system that seeks to make public the 'truth' of the trans person's gendered and sexed body" (Seid, 2014, p. 176). There is a stark contrast between film and television, where the latter has the benefit of time to develop, particularly in the amount of dialogue devoted to the reveal. Often in film, "cross-dressing is a temporary disguise rather than a symptom of a more permanent and profound identity crisis" (Phillips, 2006, p. 165). The reveals in these cases are often as simple as removing a wig. Transgender characters are not just dressing up; therefore, their reveal is riskier and more complicated.

A variety of reveal stories are told in the sample of television portrayals, ranging from difficult to nearly seamless. Transgender character Adam on *Degrassi* had transitioned socially but had not begun hormone therapy. He had transferred to Degrassi because of bullying at his old school; therefore, he has not disclosed his gender identity other than he presents as male. He is nearly outed when he accidentally drops his tampons outside of his locker. Later, Bianca, with whom Adam has been flirting, playfully touches his chest, discovering he has breasts. She ripped open his shirt and exposed his bindings (over a T-shirt) to a hallway full of students. Two boys then corner Adam in the boys' bathroom with the explicit purpose of revealing his biological sex and outing him as transgender. Exposure scenes such as this one is a violation of transgender individuals' rights because the exposers believe they have a right to see the "truth."

Cole (*The Fosters*) had socially transitioned but was still placed in a girls' group home. Within Cole's first episode, Callie accidentally walks in on him binding his breasts in the bathroom. In contrast, it is not until his fourth episode on *The Fosters* that the character Aaron voluntarily discloses to Callie (and the audience) that he is transgender. Aaron, empathizing with Callie's history of foster care and juvenile hall, tells her, "It's hard to look back on the rough stuff. I'm transgender, I get it." The discussion remains focused on Callie's problems rather than Aaron's revelation. Thus, even in his coming out as transgender, he was not defined by—nor does he define himself as—his transgender status. Although it is a dystopian tale, Sam (*Y: The Last Man*), a transgender man, struggles having survived a pandemic that has killed all living beings with a Y chromosome. Because of these circumstances, he laments that as a transgender man, he must come out again and again. "Do you have any idea what it's like out there for me? The questions I have to answer? The shit I have to explain all over again?" In contrast, Yorick, who is the lone cisgender man to survive, is mistaken for a transgender man with a few exceptions.

While it is educational to have stories of struggles that perhaps reflect reality, it is also important to include stories of easy reveals. First, the stories can model accepting behavior and positive attitudes. It can also be a hopeful message for transgender youth. In their fourth episode, Adira (*Star Trek: Discovery*) tells Paul their preference for the nonbinary pronoun "they" instead of "she." They explain, "I've never felt like a 'she' or a 'her.'" Paul, a cisgender gay man, simply smiles and moves on with the task at hand. In *Deputy*, Paula, a medical doctor who treats Bishop after a car accident, mentions a spike in Bishop's hormone levels but does not push when they insist that they are fine. Later, Bishop discloses their nonbinary gender identity. They express a great deal of relief being able to say it out loud. Paula is accepting, without questions or pushing treatment and surgical options. Bishop's coming out to their boss and coworkers are likewise met with support. In contrast, things do not go as well when Bishop discloses to their romantic partner, who breaks up with them because she is a lesbian who wants to be with a woman.

Early on in the series *Good Girls*, preteen Ben, who is still being called by his deadname, dresses in a masculine style (e.g., jaunty bowties). It is not until season two, episode five, that Ben comes out. His mother, Annie, tells him that his father and stepmother have had a new baby. She exclaims, "It's a boy!" Ben quietly reveals, "So am I." His mother is immediately accepting, hugging him and telling him she always wanted a boy. Theo (*Chilling Adventures of Sabrina*) begins "the conversation" with his father by expressing his feelings that he is more comfortable wearing a suit than a dress to a school dance. Having laid the groundwork, he continues, "Actually, Dad, I don't think I'm a girl at all. Even though I look like a girl, even though I have a girl's name, even though you've always thought of me as a girl, I'm a boy. I can't keep going on as a girl anymore. I just can't." He shares his new name, Theo, and asks if his father can take him to get a haircut. The exchange checks off three boxes in this one conversation: clothing, hair, and naming. The story has a happy ending, with his father and his close friends accepting him.

As for Casey's disclosure on *Grey's Anatomy*, showrunner Krista Vernoff stated, "The scene was rewritten more times than anything else—we wanted it exactly right." Casey tells his superior Dr. Bailey, "I'm a proud trans man, Dr. Bailey, but I'd like people to get to know me before they find out my private medical history." Dr. Bailey responds, "Of course." Vernoff notes, "We wanted the audience to get to know this character before they knew his private medical information; we wanted his disclosure to not feel like an '*A-ha!*' shock but a genuine unfolding of this character's truth when he felt safe with someone" (cited in Goldberg, 2018). His gender identity is not mentioned again in 20-plus episodes.

In *Faking It*, Shane is confused by Noah's distant behavior. Noah confesses that he was afraid to tell Shane that his parents kicked him out of the house because "they didn't accept that their daughter was actually their son." Shane replies, "It's a lot to take in but it doesn't change how I feel about you." Noah asks that Shane not share his status with anyone else. "At my old school, I was the 'trans kid.' Here I'm just Noah. I get to disclose to people when I feel comfortable." Trevor (*Shameless*), a character in his early 20s, casually discloses that he is transgender, thinking Ian already knew. Ian responds, "Holy shit, you're a chick?" Trevor laughs and corrects him that he is a transgender man. Ian asks intrusive questions such as if Trevor has a penis, to which Trevor tells him he has one, but it is made of silicone. When Trevor tells Ian that he thought Ian was nonbinary at their first meeting, Ian responds, "No, no, no. I'm normal . . . not like a dude with a vagina." Trevor snaps back, "I'm not a dude with a vagina, asshole. I'm a dude who doesn't feel like talking about his genitals." Ian chases after him, wondering what he said to upset Trevor. The exchange is grittier than other portrayals, which broaden the range of experiences.

Exposure and Vulnerability

Film reveals are often played for either comedic laughs (at the expense of the cisgender person who is fooled) or dramatic shock (at the expense of the transgender person who is either the victim or perpetrator of violence). Television takes a more nuanced approach. Very few of the recurring characters hide the fact that they are transgender. Although Max (*The L Word*) lives in a lesbian community, he does not want to be outed to his girlfriend, his boss's daughter. In one scene, he is dressed in a long-sleeved shirt and long pants, sweating profusely at a summer cookout. When his girlfriend insists that he go for a swim, he makes up an excuse that he has an ear infection and cannot go in the water. She rejects him when he finally comes out to her. In *Dead of Summer*, Drew, who is also hiding his gender identity, accidentally falls into the lake. When he gets out, he realizes his clothes are wet and clinging to his body, exposing his feminine figure. He frantically covers his chest. Mean girl Jessie throws him a towel, taunting him and calling him by his deadname. When Drew comes out to his love interest Blair, Blair walks away. Jessie and Blair eventually come around and accept Drew. Even when characters are out, there are moments when it is evident that the transition is not complete. Just as Adam's (*Degrassi*) girlfriend Becky is beginning to accept Adam as a boy, she finds a tin of tampons in his backpack. A dejected Becky says to herself, "Boys don't get their periods." Yet another reminder that Adam has not physically transitioned, an alarmed Adam drops his stand-to-pee device on the floor, splashing urine on Dave's shoes in the boys' room.

Keegan (2013) pointed to the use of the mirror scene, a classic transgender trope "where trans characters endlessly stand in front of mirrors, nude and in various stages of undress, examining themselves with a range of negative emotions running from dismay to wistful melancholy to pure disgust." Beirne (2013) called these mirror scenes "narratively unnecessary." It is another reminder that the character is still struggling. Adam (*Degrassi*) looks in the bathroom mirror as he binds, turning to the side to see if his breasts are visible. In other scenes, however, viewers could witness characters' positive reactions. For example, when the sales clerk suggests a binder for Yael (*Degrassi: Next Class*), they smile at their reflection. Likewise, Cal helps Layla (*Sex Education*) with a proper binder. Cal tells them they are glowing as they look at themselves in the mirror, laughing for the first time in the series.

In the reality genre, exposure seems more intimate than in fictional portrayals. Kyan of *Queer Eye for the Straight Guy* (2006) holds up a binding article of clothing of Miles and asks Miles to explain it. Miles describes how he has gone from sports bras to now binders to conceal his breasts. Carson, known for his bluntness, directs Miles, "Let's see what you have. Let's take the shirt off." Kyan, sensing Miles might not be okay with it, interjects, "Can we do that? Are you uncomfortable?" Miles complies. Going even further in the reboot, *Queer Eye: More Than a Makeover* (2018), the hosts are watching Skyler's top surgery at the beginning of the episode before meeting Skyler in person. They are all deeply touched by Skyler's expression as he looks down at this chest for the first time after his surgery. Critics have called out instances of "inspiration porn," such as these top surgery scenes or watching Miles give himself a shot of testosterone. Miles tells the *Queer Eye* crew that he injects himself weekly and is the one who asks the hosts if they want to see it. Kyan is very interested, while Thom becomes flustered, expressing that he would have to have to drink a bottle of vodka to inject himself.

Restroom and Changing Room Conflicts

Restrooms and locker rooms are inherently gendered spaces. These storylines are easy to understand and represent low-hanging fruit. Serano (2007) argued, "The most common expression of cissexism is denying basic privileges such as purposeful misuse of pronouns or bathroom usage." Ongoing debates about whether gender-diverse individuals should be allowed to use public facilities that align with their gender identities (see Gersen, 2016) are bringing the issue to the forefront. Usually, there is more concern with transgender women using the women's restroom than transgender men using the men's room. In a *Glee* storyline, Unique is caught using the girls' bathroom and is harassed. When she is forced to use the boys' room, she is caught and harassed again. Mr. Shu lets Unique use the faculty single-stall bathroom. Principal Sue, who holds a grudge against the glee club, installs a porta-potty with question marks all over it in the choir room. Mr. Shu negotiates a deal with Sue to allow Unique to use the faculty stall. The other glee club members accept the deal as a sign of support for Unique's transition. Early in the series *Transparent*, Moira, a transgender woman in her 60s, hesitates as she approaches the ladies' room with her daughters at the mall. Sarah signals to her that it is okay if she comes in. Overhearing Sarah call Moira "Dad," two teenage girls complain to their mother, who then confronts Moira, "Excuse me, are you a man? Because this is the ladies' restroom." Sarah notes that her father is a woman and has every right to use the women's room. The mother calls Moira a pervert and threatens to call security. After the scene, Sarah asks Moira if she is okay. Moira reluctantly replies, "I will be." A dark scene follows where Moira pulls over at a construction site and uses the porta-potty.

Michelle, one of the mothers at Dolly's (*Gypsy*) school, is gossiping with other mothers at Dolly's birthday party, "What will it be next, her own bathroom at school? I'm sorry, we can be accommodating, but I'm tired of bending over backwards. We all have our own things to worry about." Sam (*Better Things*) is called to the principal's office because her daughter Frankie was caught using the boys' restroom. The principal explains, "We have to have gender lines when it comes to the bathrooms. It's a unified policy. Even though the world has changed, we can't have unisex bathrooms in middle school." Frankie claims she does not want a unisex bathroom; she just wants to use the boys' room because her female classmates are disgusting.

Abby (*Work in Progress*), who presents as masculine but identifies as a cisgender woman, also has difficulty when using the women's restrooms. To combat prejudice and confusion, she adopts a high-pitched voice to verify her femininity. Her transgender boyfriend Chris shares that he uses an app when he travels. "Yeah, 'Refuge Restrooms.' It helps me find the nearest single stall. It saved my life when I was driving up from Kansas by myself." At a Dolly Parton concert, there is a scene in the bathroom where Abby launches into a monologue about the difficulty she has because others think she is a man. "Does anybody know how hard life is?" A transgender woman, with whom no one appears to question her presence in the women's room, comes out of a stall and states, "I've got some idea, but keep going, honey."

In the bathroom scene on *The Fosters*, an adult cisgender female stranger tells Cole he cannot use the boys' bathroom at the zoo because it would be confusing to the younger students. A young cismale bystander in the bathroom line adds, "Stay in your lane, freak." The show was clearly alluding to the bathroom debate sparked by a law in North Carolina "requiring education boards and public agencies to limit the use of sex-segregated bathrooms to people of the corresponding biological sex" (Gersen, 2016). Although the cisgender female residents from Cole's group home come to his defense during the confrontation, they are upset that they had to leave their field trip early because of the drama indirectly created by Cole. After Adam (*Degrassi*) was attacked in the boys' restroom, Principal Simpson informs Adam that he will need to use the handicap or "special needs bathroom." Theo (*Chilling Adventures of Sabrina*) uses the boys' locker room after he makes the basketball team, but the boys taunt him to "take it all off." They fill his locker with feminine hygiene products, which tumble to the floor when he opens it. In stark contrast to the basketball locker room, Michael (*Rise*) is welcomed to change with other boys in the theater dressing room. Robbie lets him know, "Yeah. That's cool." Stirring music plays in the background as Michael takes a deep breath and smiles.

Lingering Disparity in the Judicial System

Television producers use their platform to expose problems with the judicial system. In the opening scene of the *All Rise* episode "Uncommon Women and Mothers," a large man is attacking a nonbinary character, Jax, before the guards can get them out of the holding cell. The male inmate says that "she" has no place in there. Jax corrects his pronoun usage: "It's 'they,' jackass." The large man takes another swing at Jax. Jax informs their public defender Emily that they fear taking a plea deal, which will likely require prison time, stating, "I'm not tough enough for state prison. I will be killed in there." An outreach worker expresses her concern as well: "The life expectancy of a nonbinary person in this country is heartbreaking." In court, Emily asks the judge that the "they/them" pronouns be used. The judge answers, "But he looks like a 'he.'" Emily responds, "That's because you think that's what a 'he' looks like. Neither male nor female as you define it." The judge answers that it is confusing; however, although it is "going wreak havoc on the transcript," she concedes, "The court respects the defendant's identity."

Aaron gets arrested at a protest rally against ICE raids in an episode of *The Fosters*. He worries if they strip-search him, he won't be safe. He discloses his transgender status to one of the guards, who then radios there is a "situation." Aaron is released after being in solitary confinement. Aaron explains solitary is dehumanizing rather than protecting transgender inmates. In the same storyline, Callie and Aaron discuss his privilege as a white male who does not have to worry about deportation as do undocumented Latinx immigrants for whom they were protesting.

AARON: But the privilege can be instantly taken away if I'm arrested or get into a car accident.

CALLIE [discussing her friend Ximena]: She can't hide that she's Latina.

AARON: Do you think I'm hiding? It's not deceptive of me not to disclose my private medical information.

CALLIE: I'm sorry, that's not what I'm saying. People look at you and have no idea of what you have been through or how hard you've had to fight to be who you really are.

AARON: That's why people need to talk to each other, not just dismiss people they might be hurting.

Legal Documentation Hurdles

Many of the shows take on barriers presented to transgender individuals, such as documentation and identification. In *Shameless*, Trevor shies away from going to bars that might card him because his driver's license name and photo are pre-transition. When asked about getting a new one, he responds, "They make you show proof of gender confirmation surgery. So, let's all gawk at the freak show." In order to renew his DACA status, Matthew, an undocumented character on the 2020 reboot of *Party of Five*, will have to present his original birth certificate that designates his gender as female. Matthew tells his friend Lucia, "That's the only way. But that name, that's someone I never was, and I won't go back and say that's me." Casey (*Grey's Anatomy*) confesses that before he joined the staff at Grey Sloan Memorial Hospital, he was arrested for hacking into the Department of Motor Vehicles computer system to change his gender to male after they refused his request.

Karamo (*Queer Eye*, 2018) takes Skyler to have his gender marker changed on his license. Skyler tells him he needs a certificate or "surgery letter" from the hospital. The first time he went, the worker called in her supervisor, who told him to come back when he was "complete." The crew from *Queer Eye for the Straight Guy* (2006) discuss how weird it was for Miles to come out as transgender while attending an all-women's college. Miles explains, "They finally changed my sex from 'female' to 'not reported.'"

Workplace Discrimination

Coming out at work might affect one's career status, particularly if he is a transgender man or they are nonbinary. Although half of the characters in the sample were still students, careers skewed toward traditionally male occupations (e.g., doctor, firefighter, police officer, football coach). A pre-transition Max (*The L Word*) is declined a job as a computer programmer for presenting as a woman. Post-transition, he is offered the same job, making more money with the same qualifications. When his cisfeminine coworker is passed over for a promotion, Max reports the discrimination, revealing that he faced the same treatment before transitioning in order to add credibility to his coworker's claim. Nonbinary character Taylor in *Billions* experiences the privilege of not being seen as female in the male-dominated field of hedge fund investments. Taylor's temperament appears to serve them well from the boardroom to the poker table. The female characters on the show tend to be assistants or wives. Wendy, the lone female lead character, is a specialist in human behavior and dominatrix to her husband, a US attorney.

Final Thoughts

In this chapter, I demonstrate how shows are moving away from what Schenkel (2015) argued was "the rare media portrayal of transgender individuals that disproportionately focus on genitalia and surgical procedures thus dehumanizing them and fetishizing their bodies." I argue that television producers have not only increased the variety of stories being told about transmasculine characters but have included more positive models. As described above, many of these storylines share valuable information to both transgender and cisgender individuals.

It appears in this sample, once the transness of the character has been established, they are allowed to live "usual" lives, apart from their gender identity. The biggest improvement is the range of stories that were told along with nuanced journeys. They still are not perfect; however, it is definitely an improvement from past portrayals.

5 Allies and Adversaries

Acceptance of transgender individuals has increased over the years. According to Suleman (2019), polling results showed a steady three-year rise from 2016–2018 in Americans who felt comfortable with LGBTQ issues. A sharp drop occurred the following year, particularly among young adult millennials and Gen Zs who reported becoming increasingly "uncomfortable" with some of the hypotheticals presented in the survey, such as having family members or coworkers who were transgender. These findings may reflect a differentiation between "allies" (i.e., who were comfortable in all of the situations) and "detached supporters" (i.e., those whose comfort levels shifted depending on the situation) (Suleman, 2019). This chapter examines a range of characters, from allies to adversaries, under various circumstances in television series.

Allies

Of the six series that included a second transgender character, only three of them had characters that interacted with each other. Allyship is left to cisgender characters most of the time. Clare (*Degrassi*) is one of many cisfeminine allies. She plays along when Adam drops his tampons. She is understanding when he discloses his transgender status. She intervenes when she finds Adam heating a hair clip with a lighter and burning himself, comforting him, saying that he does not have to present as a girl if it does not make him happy. Sasha is Michael's (*Rise*) best friend. She is initially upset with Michael not because he came out as transgender but for not talking to her about what was going on with him. Michael tells her, "There were things I couldn't understand. How could I expect you to?" Sasha responds, "You should have given me a chance. I could have handled it. You hurt me."

Whether it is Zane (*Degrassi*), the openly gay football player; Sav (*Degrassi*), the handsome and popular student body president; or Robbie, the starting quarterback (*Rise*), cismasculine characters also act as allies.

DOI: 10.4324/9781003204404-5

Robbie, who is already struggling as a jock who is cast in the lead role in the school musical, laments "You have no idea what that just cost me" when he stands up to his fellow football players who are bullying Michael. Shane (*Faking It*) acknowledges his role in interjecting himself into Noah and his brother's fight after the brother refers to Noah by his deadname. Shane tells him, "I'm Shane and I like butting in other people's business. That's who I am. And he's Noah, he's a dude and he always has been." Later, Noah lets Shane know he can take care of himself. Shane apologizes and explains that he lost his temper hearing Noah's brother misgender him. When Shane worries about saying something dumb or insensitive, Noah answers, "You're Shane Harvey. That's pretty much a guarantee."

Two examples of adult allies are both cisgender men in positions of authority. Sheriff Bill Hollister (*Deputy*) has a reputation as a maverick, not someone expected to be an ally to his nonbinary security officer. Upon disclosing their nonbinary status, Hollister tells Bishop, "You know you don't have to be anyone but yourself with me. I might mess up sometimes . . . Live your truth." Hollister's wife, a medical doctor, is equally understanding, thanking Bishop for trusting her. She adds some educational information for the audience, "I understand there are more than two sexes. I don't understand all the layers of identity, but I do know fundamentally that not living one's truth is detrimental to your psyche."

In contrast to Hollister's rule-breaking character in *Deputy*, Fire Captain Owen Strand's (*9-1-1: Lone Star*) character is verging on savior. He is the model boss, putting together a very diverse team of firefighters in Austin, Texas. Owen has recruited Paul to work in his fire station and goes to extremes to protect Paul from the outside world. In reference to Paul's hiring, Owen's son TK warns, "If you bring in this guy, people will lose their minds." Owen simply smiles and responds, "Yep." In the pilot episode, Owen is interviewing Paul and discusses his work history. He notes that Paul has a gift for assessing situations. In a not-so-subtle way of disclosing Paul's status to the audience, he asks, "Does that have anything to do with you being trans?" Paul worries that as hard as it was in Chicago, he can't imagine what it would be like in Texas. Owen tells him, "Somewhere in this town there is a kid just like you were. Scared. Hopeless. I'd like you to show him . . . her . . . they, it's okay to be who you are. And I'll double your salary."

Micah (*The L Word: Generation Q*) struggles with speaking out when his new boss, Nat, appears overzealous about him being transgender, pointing out the gender-neutral bathrooms, for example. She declares, "It's going to be life-changing for these kids to know that a transgender therapist knows their experiences." Micah, on the other hand, feels it is demoralizing to be matched up with only transgender clients. He feels she is just checking "trans boxes." When he points out that he is capable of working with all clients, she apologizes, "I feel . . . old and dumb." She readily agrees to diversify his client base.

Fine Line Between Allies, Accomplices, and Cis Saviors

A step beyond ally, accomplices are defined as individuals who are willing to be vocal advocates (Love, 2020). Cis savior characters are those who step in to help alleviate a transgender person's suffering while putting themselves at the center. They often act as if they know more about transgender issues than the transgender character themselves, going as far as transplaining.

In the case of *Degrassi: Next Class*, there are three cisgender allies who guide Yael, a nonbinary teen, in their journey. First, a teacher observes Yael going into the boys' bathroom and asks if they are struggling. Next, a salesperson helps fit Yael with a breast binder. Third, a cisgender classmate, Lola, explains to Yael what is happening to them, getting much of her information from her favorite vlogger who identifies as genderqueer. Lola explains the different choices to Yael, who has not thought about which pronouns they prefer. "If you're not all boy or you're not all girl, why should people refer to you like you are?" A confused Yael is no match for Lola, who lectures them on gender fluidity.

Sabrina (*Chilling Adventures of Sabrina*) is an example of an accomplice. She uses her status (e.g., pretty and popular) at school to help Theo with bullies, as well as her powers as a witch to protect him. When complaining to the principal is ineffective, Sabrina takes matters into her own hands to hold the bullies accountable. Sabrina and three other witches lure the boys to the coal mines for what they think is a party. They get the boys to strip down to their underwear. Under a spell, the boys think they are passionately kissing the girls; however, they are, in fact, kissing each other. Playing on their homophobia, Sabrina takes pictures and threatens to put them up all over school if they lay a hand on Theo ever again. In season two, Theo tries out for the boys' basketball team but runs into other players and cannot make a basket. Seeing how bad Theo is at basketball and how much he wants to make the team, Sabrina put a spell on the ball. Theo starts sinking baskets and makes the team. She then gives Theo a magic rope to stop Billy from continuing to bully him, which results in Billy tripping and falling down a flight of stairs, badly injuring his leg.

Perhaps no character represents an ally/accomplice verging on savior than Callie from *The Fosters*. She represents teens in the foster care and juvenile detention system, as well as being an ally against racial discrimination and for undocumented immigrants. Her survivor instinct, intellect, and good looks make her an attractive supporter. The producers of the show are vocal in their intent to educate audiences, and Callie is the perfect catalyst. She has her boyfriend AJ and the girls in the group home as foils to lecture. While she is a strong advocate for transgender characters on the show, she, too, lacks full understanding, sometimes transplaining to others. For example, Aaron confronts Callie for sharing his status with AJ, saying, "Listen, you can't go around telling people that I'm trans . . . it's just not your story to tell. People literally get killed for being trans, so it's a really vulnerable thing to share with someone." Callie's journey of educating characters in the series continues during Callie and Aaron's visit with Aaron's parents for his father's birthday. It is immediately clear that his parents have not accepted Aaron's transition. For example, his father comments on the tattoo on Aaron's wrist, "Haven't you mutilated yourself enough?" Callie becomes visibly upset. She clarifies that Aaron is not mutilating himself but becoming who he is meant to be. Aaron later reprimands Callie, telling her that it is not her problem to fix and that he can defend himself.

The lack of multiple gender-diverse characters who appear in the same show and are allowed to interact creates a void to be filled by cis saviors. *Sex Education*, in contrast, has two nonbinary characters at their school. At one point, the headteacher pits them against each other, putting up Layla as the model nonbinary student who follows the dress code in contrast to Cal, who refuses. Cal becomes upset with Layla for failing to stand up for them. Layla later apologizes and asks Cal for assistance in a very touching scene where Cal is helping fit Layla with a binder. Cal patiently explains that binders are designed for safer chest compression than the ace bandages Layla is using, bandages that leave visible abrasions. Cal explains, "You might be tempted to wear two binders or wear a size smaller, but you shouldn't. How does it feel?" Layla laughs, "It feels so much better." A normally unemotional Cal responds, "I'm so proud of you!"

Moreover, when there is a single appearance of transgender characters in a series, cis saviors are more likely to make it all about themselves. On an episode of *Modern Family*, Mitchell excitedly tells Cam that their daughter Lily's friend Tom used to identify as Tina. Cam responds, "I wish you wouldn't have told me. You know how proud I am of my gender identificadar." As they are congratulating themselves for raising Lily, who is helping Tom through this tough time, Mitchell adds, "We deserve some kudos here, too." Cam and Mitchell hesitate when Mitchell's father Jay asks if they would accept Lily if she transitioned. Cam laments, "Are we not as open-minded as we think?" Mitchell answers, "But that's our thing, lording our tolerance over others." Kornhaber (2016) noted that Tom's appearance, although brief (under two minutes of screen time), is still small progress.

Adversaries

Twelve of the gender-diverse characters in the sample are overtly confronted by adversaries, not counting the eight instances where it is family members who are unsupportive and even abusive. The following are cases of adversarial behavior. Note that the abuse is tempered compared to film portrayals and violence against one-time-appearing transgender characters of television crime procedurals. Most of the time, allies come to their defense or the transgender characters stand up for themselves, lessening the severity of the bullying. For three transgender characters (*Degrassi*, *Chilling Adventures*, and *Dead of Summer*), their bullies even have a change of heart and become allies.

Before he is out socially, Ben is (*Good Girls*) bullied by a group of boys who are throwing food at him in the cafeteria. Ben's mother, Annie, enlists a rather hapless gang member Eddie to scare the boys. Eddie, however, goes a little overboard and threatens to break every bone in the ringleader's body. Annie later jokes about the scene to Ben's father. Harsher bullying is presented with older teen characters. Two football players ask Michael (*Rise*) intrusive questions about his transition, which escalates to pushing and shoving. Robbie, the team's quarterback, comes to Michael's defense and kicks the bullies out of his party. Star (*David Makes Man*) is called "faggot ass" and threatened by a gang member who tells him the next time he sees him, Star will be dead. Miss Elijah, a transgender woman who risks kidnapping charges by taking in Star after his family kicked him out, defends him and arranges for Star to move to another state.

Cole (*The Fosters*) is also repeatedly mistreated by some of the residents of the girls' group home where he has been placed. They consistently misgender him and say things about him such as "she is addicted to being a boy" and to stop throwing "trans-trums," When he is confronted by another boy and a middle-aged woman in the men's room line at the zoo, the girls stand up for Cole. Later, however, they are upset because Cole's actions cut their field trip short. One of the girls, Dev, goes so far as to pretend to be Cole's girlfriend but is only using him to help her get drugs. After she is exposed, she responds, "Let me tell you something, you're never going to be a boy. You're never going to be nothin' but a freak." Cole tries to stand up for himself, but he is clearly outnumbered. Callie, as discussed in the cis savior section earlier, comes to his defense time after time until he is finally moved to an LGBTQ-friendly facility.

Adult transgender characters appear to be better able to defend themselves against adversaries without the need of an ally. Kevin (*Charmed*) tells his college instructor that his roommates put a bra in his bed as a "practical joke." He refuses to file a report because, as he explains, he has dealt with worse. "I spend every day fighting, so I just want to live my life." When the Dean offers Kevin a private dorm room with its own bathroom, he responds, "My entire life, I've fought to be seen. If I let some insecure jock just shame me into the shadows, then what have I been fighting for? Dylan's just going to have to sit in his discomfort because I'm not going anywhere." When asked about his discomfort, Kevin answers, "Forcing him to see me and get to know me, that's my protest."

Taylor (*Billions*), who is wildly successful at a job as a hedge fund manager, must still deal with harassment by others. For example, Todd, Taylor's main competition at a poker tournament, twice uses the transphobic slur "that" and "that thing." After being called "cupcake," Taylor tells Todd, "I think you are trying to bully me and a bully's devastated when you stand up to him." After Taylor beats him at poker, Todd calls him a "skinny fucking freak!" and slinks away. In another scenario, an obnoxious candidate for a programming position continually refers to Taylor as "she" during the interview. Taylor remains composed, "I don't care about his insulting tone. I only care about his ability to think clearly and rationally under pressure." In another scene, Wags, the chief operating officer at the firm where Taylor works, steps in to defend them when a large Eastern European man comes into the sauna and says to Taylor, "Such disrespect. Look at you, sitting here with your tits out." Wags stands up and confronts the man: "You got a problem with my tits? Or maybe they're turning you on and that's the problem." His homophobic comeback makes the man leave. Taylor tells Wags they could have done that for themselves; however, Wags tells them he enjoys the release.

Adversaries Turned Allies

Because television appears to abhor a vacuum, as in an unresolved storyline, transphobic bullies (those who are reoccurring or minor characters) generally come around over the course of several episodes. The lesson is also taught that if the characters only can get to know a transgender person, they will change their minds. Bianca (*Degrassi*) is one of the first characters in the sample to be transformed into an ally. Initially, she enjoys being Adam's dance partner in their alternative gym class. She even flirts with him. When she playfully pushes him, her hands accidentally touch his chest. She exclaims that he is too skinny to have man boobs and rips open his shirt, exposing his binding. She outs Adam to the other students in the hallway, shouting, "What the hell? Are you a girl? I've seen you freaks on *Oprah*." In a later scene, Bianca tells Adam that he needs therapy and that if he touches her again, she will kill him. When Adam arrives at school presenting as female to pacify his mother, Bianca calls him "tranny" and "one ugly girl." Time passes and Bianca becomes romantically involved with Adam's brother Drew. She apologizes to Adam and agrees to be his dance partner again.

Not all transformations stick, in the case of Fitz, for example. Fitz and Owen follow Adam into the boys' room after hearing from Bianca about Adam's transgender identity. Fitz pressures Adam to "wiz" in the urinal and pushes Adam when he tries to leave. Owen picks up Adam over his shoulder and throws him into a glass door, which shatters. Later, however, Fitz invites Adam to sit with him at lunch. Fitz tells him, "I know we got off on the wrong foot, but I'm over it if you are." Adam, who is angry with Eli for lying to him, teams up with Fitz to make fun of Eli about wearing "guy-liner" and listening to emo music. Fitz teaches Adam how to use the clips on free weights in the school's weight room. Adam eventually gets upset with Fitz for thinking of Adam as a girl and not letting him join the boys' fight club. To show that he can compete with other boys, Adam hits Fitz in the stomach. Fitz tells him: "Say your prayers, freak. I'm finding your ass after school." At the fight, Fitz hits Eli instead. He tells Adam that he can't hit a girl, adding, "Easy, sweetheart. I could make an exception."

Adam is confronted with yet another bully in the following season, Dave, who has a problem with Adam being transgender. Although he does not physically harm or threaten Adam like Fitz and Bianca, he is still abusive. For example, he keeps referring to Adam as a "tranny." Upset that he is punished for his transphobia, Dave puts on a dress and tries to use the girls' restroom. Adam explains to Dave that being transgender is not something he can change. Dave apologizes to Adam over the school's radio station. Over time, Adam and Dave develop a strong friendship, one where Adam feels comfortable asking Dave to assess whether Adam is sufficiently hiding his chest.

Before Theo's transition in season one of *Chilling Adventures of Sabrina*, Billy and Carl bully Theo because of his androgynous appearance. Billy calls him a "dyke." Theo rushes Billy, who then punches Theo in the face. The bullies laugh and run away. To get Billy to stop, Sabrina offers Theo a magic rope. Instead of just tripping him, the rope causes Billy to fall down the stairs. His leg is clearly broken and bleeding. Later, at the school dance, Billy approaches Theo on crutches and tells Theo his new short haircut "looks bad-ass." He apologizes for "being such a dick." Billy explains that he is tired of bad things happening to him.

When Jessie (*Dead of Summer*) discovers Drew is transgender, she begins to make derogatory remarks, describing him as a "freak" and calling him by his deadname. Drew directs her not to say anything, going so far as to blackmail her with a letter showing she lied on her job application for the camp counselor position. In retaliation, Jessie tells Drew that she has been filming him in the shower. Fearing Jessie's threats to out him, Drew packs up and leaves the camp. Jessie finds him at the bus station. She tells him she lied about videotaping him. He admits he was never going to tell the other counselors about the letter. She concludes that they are kind of the same and that they are both scared of being who they are. Drew tells her he is not trying to hide who he is; he is trying to be who he is. She tells him she hopes he comes back. They eventually make up and become allies.

Michael (*Mistresses*) and April begin a flirtation when they first meet. After Michael comes out as transgender, April denies her initial attraction to him. She adds that he is no longer a threat to her relationship with her boyfriend because she would never date a transgender person, upsetting him. Michael yells at her to get out of his house. April's mother goes even further with her transphobic comments. She tells April, "Transgender? And you knew it and still worked with him? What is the world coming to? Why do these people think they can flaunt themselves in front of everybody and we all have to accept it? My opinion is that it's unnatural." It is not until April hears her mother's bigotry that she realizes the harm she has done to Michael and apologizes.

Sue Silvester from the series *Glee* is an interesting case study of a character who is both ally and adversary: a mix of insensitivity, sometimes even cruel, yet other times compassionate. As principal, Sue pushes two students to encourage Unique, a transfeminine character from McKinley High's rival glee club Vocal Adrenaline, to wear a dress and heels while performing. Sue reasons that the transphobic judges will be compelled to vote against the team because of Unique. Handing Kurt and Mercedes a pair of heels, Sue instructs them to get Unique to "cram his ham hocks into these platoons at regionals." When Unique later transfers to McKinley High, Sue refuses to let her use the faculty bathroom after being bullied in the girls' and boys' rooms. Instead, she installs a porta-potty covered with question marks in the middle of the choir room. Sandercock (2015) concluded that the satire and dark humor of *Glee*, particularly regarding the treatment of the transfeminine character Unique, is problematic.

Sue is also abusive to Coach Beiste, who initially presents as a woman. Sue claims that female football coaches are sins against nature. When Coach Beiste tells Sue about his impending transition, she responds, "When you think about it, it's not that big of a stretch." In other ways, Sue shows compassion toward Coach Beiste, telling him his job will be waiting if he wishes to return after his surgery. She also chases out a group of students who vandalize and write "tranny" on his car. She tells him she has taken steps to battle the scourge of cisnormativity and transmisogyny, although these are terms she had never heard of until she did a "quick Wikipedia search." Her behavior continues to be inconsistent: she is both a bully and an advocate for comic effect. Immediately after announcing that McKinley is a fully gender-fluid high school, she adds, "All right, now if you'll excuse me, out of the corner of my eye, I see fatty who could use a good, healthy fat-shaming." She is set up as an equal opportunity insulter, even though she declares she has always been vocal about her opposition to bullying. She is survival-of-the-fittest in a tracksuit, any empathy potentially making her look weak. What is likely most impactful is the comic framing of her character, unlike the other adversaries described in this section. The joke work signals the audience not to take her words and actions seriously.

Romantic Partners and Navigating Relationships

A major part of what it means to be a transgender ally or adversary is how the characters navigate romantic relationships and dating challenges. Blair and Hoskin (2019) found only about 3% of heterosexual men and women said they would date a transgender person versus almost 90% of transgender or nonbinary individuals. The recurring characters in my television sample experience an array of successful and unsuccessful romantic relationships. The advantage of television over film is that there is more screen time available to explore the nuances in some of these relationships. In contrast to shocking reveals of transgender characters in films such as *The Crying Game* and *Boys Don't Cry*, these television shows take a more measured exploration of what happens when a character's gender identity is shared or exposed. Unlike crime shows, which often present single-episode transgender individuals as devious or even sex workers, most of the reoccurring transgender characters in my sample appear to be treated with respect.

Out of the 44 transgender characters in my sample, 28 were shown to be in some sort of romantic relationship, which is a positive sign that transgender characters are deserving of love. At times, however, these relationships are presented as messy and in need of special negotiations, unlike those between two cisgender individuals. Four transgender characters were rejected by the other party immediately after their reveal. All five relationships that clearly started before the characters transitioned later failed. The outcomes demonstrate that it is generally riskier for the transgender character, with the cisgender party having more of the power to accept, redefine, or reject the relationship.

The *Degrassi* franchise, which dates back to the 1980s, is based on a great many dating pairings; therefore, it is not unusual that Adam would have multiple love interests. Adam initially had a crush on Bianca, who outed and threatened him. He then turns his attention toward Katie. Although it appears that she is flirting with him, it quickly becomes clear that she is not interested in him in "that way." While the decisions to break up are mostly made by the nontransgender person, there are exceptions. After experiencing a series of unrequited loves, Adam (*Degrassi*) begins a relationship with Fiona. Fiona, who identifies as bisexual, tells Adam that it does not matter that he is transgender. However, when she tells him that she likes how he is the "best of both worlds" because he is "boyish and girlish," Adam breaks up with her because he rejects his feminine side and wants to be seen only as a boy. Adam's one truly successful relationship is with a conservative Christian, cisgender girl who initially had issues dating him. At one point, she must also contend with the shock at finding his tampons, a reminder that he has only socially transitioned. Becky eventually overcomes her religious background and conservative parents to accept Adam. She rationalizes, "Adam's a boy. I wouldn't have feelings for him if he weren't." Adam finds happiness with Becky, only to die in a car accident while trying to text her while driving.

The Fosters devotes significant screen time to both Cole's and Aaron's relationships. Cole is the first to have a crush on Callie. He misinterprets her platonic offer to go with him to an alternative prom as romantic. He becomes upset when she pulls away as he moves in to kiss her. She tries to explain that her rejection is not because he is transgender but because she only likes him as a friend. Callie later dates Aaron, demonstrating that she is okay dating a transgender person. She ultimately shows that it does not make her transphobic if she is not attracted to a specific transgender person. After being rejected by Dev and Callie, Cole worries he will never be loved that way. Although she does not appear on screen, Cole later talks about having a girlfriend and how she makes him feel manly.

In contrast to her platonic relationship with Cole, Callie is attracted to Aaron. She kisses him before she is aware that he is transgender and is still attracted to him after he comes out to her. *The Fosters* promoted Elliot Fletcher, the actor playing Aaron, as a teen heartthrob (Mackie, 2016) in a leather jacket and riding a motorcycle. Callie's boyfriend AJ becomes jealous of Aaron's flirtation with Callie. After he finds out Aaron is transgender, AJ expresses that he no longer feels threatened by Aaron. Callie scolds him, "That's a very ignorant thing to say. Aaron is no less of a man than you are. And just cause he's trans, that would never stop me from seeing him." Callie and Aaron eventually begin dating after she and AJ break up.

Overall, younger characters in my sample appear more open to dating transgender individuals. In the final episode *Rise*, like every good rom-com, teen best friends Michael and Sasha kiss. In contrast, Josie (*9-1-1: Lonestar*), who is a cisgender woman in her 30s, calls Paul the "man of her dreams" but cannot get past his transgender status after he comes out to her. Paul makes an interesting comment about sticking to using dating apps, where he can screen out women who are not willing to date a transgender man. Younger transgender male characters appear to also rebound faster after rejection. Matthew (*Party of Five*), who appears to be in his late teens, explains that even though his conversation with a girl did not go well, one he describes as clumsy and embarrassing, he is excited that he could actually flirt with a girl.

Former lesbian relationships with transitioning male characters appear to present a different challenge for cisgender women. Jenny is initially excited about participating in Max's (*The L Word*) transition and even offers to help with Max's hormone injections. Their relationship is damaged as Max becomes more aggressive, seemingly because of the testosterone. Ultimately, Jenny breaks up with him because she is a lesbian and Max is a man. Jake (*Tales of the City*) and Margot were dating before his transition as well. She tells her friend that Jakes says they "are queer now;" however, she misses being a lesbian. He gets upset when Margot makes a reference to "when we were lesbians." He corrects her, "You mean, when I was pre-transition." When the subject of having children is broached, Jake asks, "Why is it so crazy to ask for a second to breathe while I figure out my body before we make a person." Margot snaps back, "Why is it about your body? Why not my body and the words I want to use and how you can't give a shit about how shitty it makes me feel?" Margot tells him that she knows she is not allowed to, but she misses him pre-transition. Jake feels hurt but wants to try working on their relationship. Margot is not able to continue with the relationship and breaks it off. Michael (*Mistresses*) shares with April that his wife filed for divorce after he transitioned. He explains, "I honestly thought our relationship might be enough for me to be happy, but as time went on, I needed more. I need to live fully as myself. She understood at first. But after a while, I think it was too much for her."

Cismasculine gay characters are shown as accepting of transgender partners, although often after struggling with their partner's gender identity reveals. Shane (*Faking It*) eventually gets over his discomfort with Noah's transgender identity, although he half-jokingly fears the gay community will "rip up his gay card" if he dates a transgender man. Blair (*Dead of Summer*) also hesitates at first but comes to see Drew as a man, telling him, "When you first came here, I thought you were the hottest guy I'd ever seen. And I still do." Ian (*Shameless*) struggles at first with dating Trevor. Trevor gets frustrated, telling Ian, "I'm a dude who doesn't feel like talking about his genitals." Trevor informs him, "Don't do me any favors. I can fuck any guy here. I don't need your cisgender ass." They end up dating; however, their relationship does not last not because Trevor is transgender but because of Ian's relationship with an old boyfriend. Micah (*The L Word: Generation Q*) tells Jose that he has not met a lot of people "who don't squint and try to imagine what I used to look like." Jose accepts him as he is, but of course, in true dramatic fashion, Micah discovers Jose is married.

Nonbinary characters appear to be more in control of their relationships with both cismasculine and cisfeminine partners than the transmasculine characters. At first, Joey (*Good Trouble*) and Alice continue their relationship after Joey comes out as nonbinary. Over time, however, Joey is offended that Alice is joking about Joey's pronouns in her stand-up act. Alice, thinking she is empathizing with Joey, tells them she doesn't know who she is either. Joey retorts they know who they are and breaks up with Alice, who appears not to "get" who Joey is. *Sex Education* goes much more in-depth, explaining nuances of nonbinary relationships further than other series. As they are growing closer, Cal explains to Jackson, "If this was going to become more serious, you'd be in a queer relationship. Is that okay with you?" Jackson, discussing the issues with his lesbian mother, concludes that he is not queer. Cal insists that they just be friends. Jackson tries to reason with them, "I thought you were all about breaking out of boxes. So, what does it matter if I'm queer or if I'm not?" Cal responds that because they are not a girl, they worry that he still sees them as one. Jackson, still not getting it, tells them he is open and willing to learn. Cal explains, "Here's the thing. I'm still figuring out so much shit about myself. I can't carry you, too. And I still want to have fun when I can because I feel so heavy all the time." Yael's (*Degrassi: Next Class*) boyfriend Hunter is struggling with changes in their gender presentation (e.g., not shaving their legs and underarms). Hunter's friend Vijay tries to explain, "Yael is still the same person on the inside. And, if you loved that person before, why can't you love them now?" Hunter says he wants Yael to be happy, but this is too much for him. Faced with a decision to be true to themself or appease Hunter, Yael declares, "This is me. I guess if he loves me, he'll come around. But I'm not going back. Not for him. Not for anyone."

Bishop's (*Deputy*) girlfriend Genevieve goes through a range of emotions after Bishop discloses their nonbinary identity, as illustrated in the following exchange:

BISHOP: Actually, you assumed I was a woman, and in what should come as no surprise, I'm a little more complicated than that. Look, Gen. This is me finally living my truth. Being the most authentic version of myself. And I need you to understand that.

GEN: I do, I just feel like I don't know who you are anymore.

BISHOP: I'm the same person you fell in love with. I haven't changed. I'm still me. I'm just a clearer version of me.

GEN: I need time to process this . . . I'm a lesbian. A woman who likes women. And if you're not a woman, what does that mean for me? For us?

BISHOP: I can't tell you what that means for you, but for us, I know that I have to bring my whole self to this relationship.

GEN: Did you know when you moved here you were nonbinary?

BISHOP: I didn't have a term for it, but I knew that something about me was different. But that doesn't change how I feel about you. I know we can get through this. But you don't.

GEN: I don't know if I can.

Conversations such as these portray more of the nuance of relationships pre- and post-transition. Although they break up, Bishop later finds happiness with someone who accepts them as nonbinary.

There were two characters who did not fit in the mold of traditional relationships. Abby (*Work in Progress*) defines herself as a queer dyke, and therefore, as the character explains, she has no issues with Chris identifying as a transgender man. There are some challenges as she still must continuously explain their relationship to her friends and family. Ali (*Transparent*), a cisgender woman who appears to be struggling with her bisexuality, has an odd relationship with a transgender man. He later accuses her of being a "chaser," someone who likes transgender people because they are transgender. These variations are important in terms of showing the legitimacy and positive and negative aspects of alternative relationships.

Negotiating Sex

Television series include a distinct element of voyeurism—particularly with how cisgender partners deal with a transgender body. As they start to have sex, Ian (*Shameless*) pauses, then says, "I don't know how to do this." Trevor responds, "I'll show you." They begin to laugh hysterically when they realize the difficulty they are having is because they are both tops. Hassan, a cisgender gay man Micah (*The L Word: Generation Q*) met on Grindr, asks, "I've never been with a trans guy. What should I do?" Chris (*Work in Progress*) discloses to Abby that he does not like to have his chest touched since he has not been able to afford chest masculinization surgery. Shows like *The Fosters* tend to focus more on the relationship than just sex. As Callie and Aaron's relationship heats up, she asks Cole for advice about being intimate with a transgender man. Cole tells her he likes it when his girlfriend comments on how masculine he is. Aaron asks why she is being so weird when she tells him "You're so strong" and "I love your stubble." Callie fears that she will hurt his feelings while he gets upset with her for making things so complicated. Aaron confesses that he is not ready for them to have sex because it makes him feel vulnerable, and he wants to be sure he can trust her. In contrast to the previous examples, Oscar (*Billions*) appears to have no issues with Taylor being nonbinary. He never once misgenders them and never enquires about Taylor's gender or sexual preferences.

Family Dynamics

Poole's (2017) article "Towards a Queer Futurity: New Trans Television" notes that factors such as generational conflicts and family constellations play an important role in portrayals. In my sample, family dynamics appear in many of the narratives, ranging from supporting to rejecting and the processing in between. Eleven transgender characters have supportive families, eight unsupportive, and three mixed, while 22 make no reference to family members' reactions to their transitions.

Supportive

Of the families that either appeared in the series or were at least mentioned, a majority were supportive of the transgender character. On one end of the acceptance spectrum, Michael's (*Rise*) family fully embraced his transition, as discussed in the following dialogue:

SASHA: Let me guess, [your sister] drove 200 miles from Kenyon College that very night, bought you a tub of ice cream. You stayed up all night listening to lame Sam Smith songs and weeping in each other's arms. And your parents—your parents were like, "Michael. We love the name Michael. We love you no matter what your name is, what your gender is. You are our perfect angel." Tell me I didn't nail it.

MICHAEL: Pretty much word-for-word.

Annie (*Good Girls*) is very supportive of her transgender son Ben. His dad gets onboard fairly quickly, while his stepmother is a bit neurotic and overcompensates by repeating his chosen name over and over. Theo's (*Chilling Adventures of Sabrina*) father had experience with what he calls his brother's "proclivities." He explains that when they were young, Jesse was beaten by their father for wearing their mother's dresses. When it came time for Theo to come out, his father paused ever so slightly and then agreed to take Theo to get a new haircut as a symbol of his acceptance.

In the case of *Gypsy*, the mothers at Dolly's school are more passive-aggressive than directly abusive. When Dolly's mother Jean overhears one of the mothers, Michelle, complaining about having to accommodate gender-diverse students, she confronts Michelle. "I'm not going to play this game anymore and I'm not going to pretend that this is acceptable, because it's not. We're all just lying all the time by pretending to be friends and not buying into the politics . . . You're the reason why my little girl has to be scared of being judged."

For transgender actor Blue Chapman's (who plays JJ) mother, it was important that *Council of Dads* included a supportive family. JJ's parents and siblings were not only tolerant but fully accepting of his identity. They often spoke out against misgendering and transphobic comments. JJ's oldest sister Luly is a particularly staunch advocate. From a bathroom stall, Luly overhears some women from her mother-in-law's church saying transphobic things about JJ. Luly scolds them and tells her husband, Evan. Although Evan tells her not to take it personally, Luly states that she cannot look the other way. JJ's other siblings take his gender identity in stride. Unlike other shows with young characters, such as *Degrassi*, they are not confronted with peer bullying as none of the action takes place at JJ's school. Adam's stepbrother Drew has transferred to Degrassi High with Adam in order to escape transphobic bullying at their old school. When Drew sees Adam is being targeted again, he gets upset and tries to fight the bully, vowing not to let anyone hurt or touch Adam again. While Drew supports Adam, his allyship is not without consequences. Unlike other characters, Adam's gender identity affects Drew in terms of having to switch schools and becoming a target for bullies by association.

Unsupportive

An estimated 70,000 transgender youth lack secure housing in the US (Holder, 2019). Nationally, an estimated 40% of unhoused youth in the US identify as LGBTQ, nearly a quarter of whom identify as transgender and nonbinary. Some of the television portrayals reflect reality in that parents often kick their transgender children out of the house when they come out. After Cole's (*Fosters*) parents kicked him out of the house, he reports doing what he had to do to survive, such as stealing and engaging in sex work. Even when he is hospitalized after a bad reaction to street testosterone, his parents still do not come to see him. Noah (*Faking It*) was likewise kicked out of the house when he came out as transgender. When his brother Brody shows up to see him, he asks Noah, "What the hell have you done to yourself?" He tells Noah that their parents agreed to let him come home if he goes back to presenting as a girl. Noah rejects the offer, after which Brody calls Noah by his deadname and tells him that he and his boyfriend are freaks. Max's (*The L Word*) sister Sioban calls him disgusting, adding, "Mom told me on her deathbed that she thought you should've been born a boy. But look at you. You're a freak now. I'm glad she's not alive to actually see it." What these cases and nearly all these bad parents and siblings have in common is that they are one-appearance or, at most, minor characters if they appear on screen at all (i.e., the transgender characters simply recount past abuse). Television shows in this sample, however, tend not to dwell on the abusive interactions with family members.

Drew's (*Dead of Summer*) mother rejects, accepts, and then rejects Drew. She first refuses to accept Drew's gender identity throughout his childhood. After seeing how happy he is presenting as male, she tells him, "I saw you. I saw you, Drew. I know that now. You are a boy. You *are* a boy. I'm sorry." However, his mother ends up leaving, explaining in a note that she cannot accept that her daughter was not real and that seeing Drew every day is a reminder of what she lost.

Struggling to Support

Familial characters' struggles add to the conflict of television dramas. At the same time, exploring how family members reach acceptance is an important lesson for viewers. Adam's (*Degrassi*) mother is generally supportive but is still adjusting to his transition. Early on, she admits that she still sees Adam as a girl and often stumbles with using the correct pronouns. Over time, she tells him that she is proud of the man he is becoming and relents to his requests to start talking to a doctor about taking testosterone. Although she appears to accept his choices, Jake (*Tales of the City*) admits his mother breaks a hundred "trans rules" every time she texts him. Jake's father also appears to be trying to accept him. Jake's uncle Mando, on the other hand, is dismissive and questions Jake's masculinity. When Jake refuses a beer, Mando asks if he wants a wine cooler, implying something more feminine. Micah's (*The L Word: Generation Q*) mother repeatedly makes errors as well. When first meeting Micah's boyfriend Jose, she tells him that Micah was crafty, ever since "he was a little girl." She shows Jose pictures of Micah in a little white dress before his transition. Micah finally raises his voice, telling her to stop. His mother realizes that although she is trying, it is not good enough, but she promises to do better.

While Aaron's (*The Fosters*) mother is working on accepting his transition, Aaron's father is passive-aggressive, making jokes and accusing Aaron of mutilating his body. While there is no resolution with his father by the end of the episode in which they appear, his mother places an updated photograph of him along with the other family photos on the fireplace mantle. She laments, even doing so using the incorrect pronoun, "I think of all the pain that I caused her, every time I put her in a dress or take ballet, join the Girl Scouts. Things I thought would make her happy. I must have made her life so hard." Results of the sample show that it is more common for mothers to be accepting and defend their transgender children from unsupportive or struggling fathers.

After Max's (*The L Word*) mother dies, Max goes back to his hometown for the funeral. His father, who fits Suleman's (2019) concept of a detached supporter, gives Max his mother's charm bracelet and even refers to Max as "son." At the wake, however, he appears embarrassed of Max and introduces him to everyone as his wife's cousin's son from California rather than as his own son whom he formally considered his daughter. Max ends up watching the burial off to the side where he cannot easily be seen. Taylor (*Billions*) is impatient with his father's misgendering and use of air quotes when using their preferred pronouns. His father concedes, "Hey, kid, you know I don't think that 'woke' stuff is all worthless or for idiots just because I'm not good at it, right? I know it matters."

Generational differences are further highlighted in family supportiveness. On *9-1-1*: *Lone Star*, Paul explains to his coworkers that his mother accepts him but that he and his sister Naomi have not been on speaking terms ever since he transitioned. When they stop in for a visit, Paul accuses Naomi of never having dealt with who he is. She explains that she does not care that Paul is transgender, only that he left home when she was only nine years old, and nobody explained to her why. "She left, and you came back, and it felt to me like you killed her. So no, P. It's you who never dealt with me. You say I'm mad because you left. No. I'm mad because she did. And she never said goodbye." Paul admits he did not consider what she was going through and the two make up.

In the following cases, it is grandparents or other older characters who have issues. In *Council of Dads*, JJ's grandmother dresses him as a girl for his father's funeral, explaining that she thought it would make everything easier. Robin, JJ's mother, accuses her mother of only making things easier for herself. The grandmother tries to defend herself, "You have to understand, I'm her grandma. And I love her, and she's so young." When she later trips up and misgenders JJ, she recalls that she has been told that when she does that, not to make a big deal about it, apologize, and move on. Six-year-old JJ simply shrugs. Dolly's (*Gypsy*) grandmother has similar issues with acceptance. She makes passive-aggressive comments about the shortness of Dolly's hair and Dolly's choice to bow instead of curtsey after Dolly's performance as Peter Pan. Adam's (*Degrassi*) mother pressures Adam to present as a girl for his grandmother to make things "easier." His grandmother is coming to dinner, and his mother tells Adam that it would be nice if "Gracie" could join them. Adam reminds her that "Gracie" is gone and that he is not going to play dress-up for anyone. His mother then tells him not to come to dinner if he intends to introduce his grandmother to "Adam." Adam does appear at dinner, presenting as a girl. Adam announces that he has something to say, but because of his mother's request not to say anything, he changes his mind, leaving his grandmother in what appears to be peaceful ignorance.

Educators: Woke, Unwoke, and Nearly Woke

Many of these shows feature adolescents and teens; therefore, scenes often take place at school. Educators in media portrayals can be idealized, always saying the right thing at the right time. A cisfeminine teacher checks in with Yael (*Degrassi: Next Class*) after noticing some changes in Yael. She wants to make sure the school is supporting them (e.g., using a different bathroom or using a different pronoun). She lets Yael know, "Questioning your gender identity can come with depression and anxiety, but you don't have to go through it alone. This school has had other transgender students before . . . we just want to know so that we can help." In the pilot episode of *Rise*, Mr. Mazzushelli (or Mr. Mazzu as he is affectionately called) represents that model teacher who is sensitive and supportive. He asks Michael, a transitioning student, what he would like to be called after seeing Michael has written "Margaret (Michael) Hallowell" on the audition sign-up sheet. When he answers, "Michael," Mr. Mazzu quietly responds, "Beautiful."

Teachers and principals are also portrayed as "woke" allies, well-meaning but hindered by school system rules and procedures. For example, the principal on *Better Things* demonstrates some sympathy but takes no action. She states, "We have to have gender lines when it comes to the bathrooms. It's a unified policy. Even though the world has changed, we can't have unisex bathrooms in middle school." After Adam (*Degrassi*) was thrown into a glass door, his mother demands that Adam be transferred to another school. Principal Simpson suspends the bullies and makes accommodations in order to keep Adam safe. These well-meaning accommodations turn out to be burdensome to Adam. In addition to being assigned a teacher to walk him to class, Adam will need to use the handicapp bathroom.

More infrequent is the unsupportive educator. The headteacher on *Sex Education* first appears progressive; however, her ambitions get in the way. In order to restore the school's reputation, she requires gender-specific school uniforms. Cal, a nonbinary student, is punished for noncompliance. She tells Cal if they are not going to wear the skirt uniform, they at least have to wear pants that fit more to their body. She points to another nonbinary student who is uniform compliant. Cal responds, "So Layla's a good NB, and I'm a bad one. Is that right?" She tells Cal they can talk but only when Cal wears the "correct" uniform to school.

Sabrina (*Chilling Adventures of Sabrina*) goes to Principal Hawthorne to report the school's football players for pulling up Theo's (pre-transition) shirt because they wanted to see whether he is "a boy or a girl." Principal Hawthorne shows little sympathy in terms of Theo's sexual identity dilemma, suggesting he find another school rather than punishing the bullies. Shortly thereafter, he is replaced with Principal Wardwell (who is more supportive but has her own agenda via the storyline of witches). The boys' basketball coach also represents old-school misogyny and transphobia. While he stops the fighting between Theo and the bullies in the gym, he refuses to allow Theo to try out for the boys' team because he does not allow "girls." Principal Wardwell informs the coach that it is unacceptable to refuse tryouts, and there shall be absolutely no gender discrimination at Baxter High. The coach reluctantly agrees, disparagingly calling Theo "four-foot nothing."

Religious Adversaries

Examples of religious intolerance emerged as a subcategory of adversarial characteristics. As discussed earlier, Luly (*Council of Dads*) gets upset with her husband for not supporting her when a pair of church ladies disparage her transgender brother. "This isn't just stupid stuff. And these people are your mom's church. Your church that you keep telling me played such an important role in how you grew up. And you wonder why I don't come every Sunday with you guys because these people are not my people." In another instance, April's (*Mistresses*) mother goes on a transphobic rant when she learns Michael is transgender. April tells her, "I thought you raised me to be tolerant of others." Her mother replies, "I raised you to be a proud, Black, Christian woman. Not running around with people who have none of the values you grew up with."

Becky (*Degrassi*) comes from an extremely religious family. She leads a protest of the school's gender-bending version of *Romeo and Juliette* renamed *Romeo and Jules*, which she calls a "blasphemous musical that normalizes alternative lifestyles." As she develops feelings for Adam, she worries that he will turn her gay. Her friend Jenna explains that Adam is not gay and that he is not a girl who likes girls but rather a boy who likes girls. Becky warms to the idea as she gets to know Adam. At one point, she decides she does not want to keep Adam a secret, so she tells her parents that he is transgender. While at first seeming to accept Adam, Becky's father hands him a pamphlet about conversion therapy in order to "fix" him. Becky's mother puts pressure on her, asking if she is ready to give up her relationship with God to be with Adam. Becky relents to her parents' wishes. She tells Adam that she cannot choose him over her family and her faith; therefore, she is going to try therapy herself. When she returns from conversion camp, she tells Adam, "It's not working. The therapy. It doesn't cure feelings. Sitting there every day only reminds me that I like boys, and you're a boy . . . and no therapy or prayer will ever change that." Becky stands up to her father, declaring her love for Adam. As with other storylines, the parents disappear from the remaining episodes, and the issue is never fully resolved.

A religious theme also emerges from the reality show *Strut*. Laith Ashley's mother shares her struggles to accept her son because of her religion. By accepting him, she thinks she is also sinning. Laith confronts her, "You say it's a sin and I'm going to hell." His mother answers, "I don't say that. My Bible says that." He tells her, "Do you know how many times I threw myself on the floor and prayed so I can change? Thinking that if I die, I'll go straight to hell because of who I am?" His mother tells him that only God can change that part of his life. She ultimately wants him to be happy. By the end of the six-episode series, she calls Laith her "son," although it is unclear where she stands in terms of her religion.

Final Thoughts

A common strategy used by television producers and writers is to create a dichotomy of characters, as either allies or adversaries, for dramatic effect. Transphobic straw persons are set up (most likely one-time characters) so that allies (most likely major characters) can come to the rescue, sometimes crossing the line into cis savior territory, especially in earlier series. Parents who are cast as either supportive or unsupportive follow a distinct pattern. Main characters tend to accept their gender-diverse children, while those who reject their children are nearly always one-appearance characters. Several lessons can be learned from these portrayals. According to the social learning theory, media can offer audience members models for acceptance. The shows in my sample rewarded empathetic cisgender allies. While there are cases of bullying, especially in the shows targeting youth audiences, the shows are likely to teach accountability and redemption. In other words, many characters "learn their lesson" and come around to not just tolerate but accept transgender characters.

Afterword

Scholars in the field of communication and mass media have long argued that television educates and shapes culture (Siebler, 2010). Increased exposure to transgender characters, especially those who are treated as respected members of the cast, can challenge stereotypes (see Capuzza & Spencer, 2017). My goal here was to look critically at transgender representation from the perspective of a mainstream television audience, particularly viewers with no direct awareness of individuals whose gender varies from that assigned to them at birth. The importance of this type of analysis cannot be understated, especially in a highly volatile political climate that targets LGBTQ individuals.

Serano (2016) noted, "While a decade is not a huge amount of time in the grand scheme of things, it certainly feels like a lifetime ago when it comes to public understandings and discussions about transgender people." In the half decade since, I argue even more changes have occurred. GLAAD president and CEO Sarah Kate Ellis noted, "Hollywood changed how Americans understand gay and lesbian lives, and TV is starting to do the same for transgender people with authentic transgender portrayals" (cited in Stedman, 2018). Early transgender television roles often reflected troubling trends found in film, such as using gender variance as a plot device and relying on the novelty of transgenderism and shocking reveals. For example, older situation comedies often include transfeminine characters reappearing post-transition to surprise an unsuspecting, semi-transphobic friend. Crime dramas are fond of portraying one-off characters, mostly transgender women, as victims of "trans panic" (i.e., blaming the victims for the violence because they deceived the perpetrators) assaults. Creating accurate and respectful portrayals often depends on giving characters enough screen time to develop as individuals beyond their gender identity. I found a stark contrast between dramas that incorporate transgender characters as part of the community and situation comedies that offer up transgender characters as the butt of the joke. The significant percentages of episodes in which transgender characters appear in my sample indicate that they are getting far better treatment currently than in the past. I found 20 out of 44 transgender characters appear in over half of the episodes of the series' runs, with 11 of them appearing in 90% to 100% of the episodes. Only nine characters who meet the three-episode minimum appear in less than 10% of the episodes.

According to GLAAD, too few shows do too much of the work of television's LGBTQ representation (cited in Mitovich, 2021). In terms of transmasculine characters, my sample shows a relatively equal distribution among broadcast networks (11 shows with 12 characters), cable networks (15 shows with 18 characters), and streaming services (12 shows with 14 characters). The highest representations appear on the basic cable network Freeform (four shows with six characters), the premium cable channel Showtime (six shows with seven characters), and the streaming service Netflix (eight shows with nine characters). There is at least one representation on each of the five broadcast networks (see Appendix B).

In my sample, early transmasculine depictions include tropes such as Max (*The L Word*) experiencing "roid rage" in 2006 and Cole (*The Fosters*) ending up in the emergency room after taking street testosterone in 2014. Much of the mid-airing representation of masculinity expression focused on short haircuts and chest binding. More contemporary portrayals were complex and varied, expanding beyond discussions of genitalia, gender affirmation surgery, and body dysphoria. Although hormone therapy and chest masculinization surgery were often discussed, shows demonstrated that identifying as transgender is not solely dependent upon physical appearance. While not perfect, producers spent additional screen time on representations beyond gender binaries, gradually including more gender-questioning and gender-fluid characters.

The results of this study, which found a reduction in wrong body tropes and gender dysphoric stereotypes over time, make a case for advances in the "respecting" transgender individuals, as outlined in Clark's (1969) fourth stage of media representation for social groups. Clark argued that groups often go through stages from invisibility and ridicule to respect. Similarly, Suzanne Danuta Walters explained the difference between simply tolerating such characters and fully accepting them in her book *The Tolerance Trap* (2014). She argued, "Being seen in popular culture is often mistaken as the sure sign of social inclusion" (p. 154). She further noted that tolerance falls short of the goal of acceptance. Television versions of tolerance include educators offering students the use of a separate bathroom in the nurse's office or parents allowing sons or daughters to present as themselves in private but insisting they "change back" to their gender assigned at birth for public events or for grandparents who "wouldn't understand." Once shows advance past the obligatory backstory (e.g., when did the character know they were transgender) and discussions of what happens in the transition process (e.g., focus on surgery or medical treatment), they move closer to acceptance.

Maura Keisling of the National Center for Transgender Equality described media portrayals as moving from something new and quirky to becoming more normalized over time (cited in Ulaby, 2014). This goal of normalization, or becoming unremarkable, was explored in Andre Cavalcante's (2018) *Struggling for Ordinary: Media and Transgender Belonging in Everyday Life*, a collection of interviews. The book described how transgender individuals "made their way toward a sense of ordinary life by integrating available media into their everyday experiences." The inclusion of not one but two transmasculine characters played by transgender actors in the fictional show *The Fosters* was a significant step toward ordinary. Tom Phelan, who played Cole, stated, "I think there was the prerequisite capital T transgender storyline, but after that I got to have a love interest, and be funny, and have fun, and have friends, and go to the beach. That's the sort of story I think is the most important. Just normal people, doing people things" (cited in Schultz, 2016). Elliot Fletcher, who played Aaron on the show, added, "The future of Hollywood that I want to see for trans people—normal, which is a loaded term to begin with, but trans people need to be normalized. I want there to be a movie starring a trans man or transmasculine person where they don't go on hormones and they don't have surgery because that's a really legitimate trans experience" (cited in Whitney, 2017). The characters show transgender individuals can be regular cast members involved in storylines unrelated to their gender identity. They can help solve crimes, date pretty cisgender girls, and attend birthday parties. These portrayals allow audience members to see that while being transgender is part of who they are, it does not wholly define them. Whoopie Goldberg, an executive producer on the reality series about a transgender modeling agency *Strut*, suggested, "Maybe if we realize that transgender people have moms and dads and boyfriends, that we can be kinder when we are with them" (cited in Miller, 2016).

In addition to more voices and more representation, character portrayals should be expanded beyond their struggles. Marzano-Lesnevich (2021) called for writers to create a world in which transgender youth do not just endure but thrive. In reparative narratives, transgender character storylines have happy endings. Sandercock (2015) also called for young transgender characters not to be limited to negative experiences such as discrimination and assaults but instead be included in positive portrayals such as friendship and romance. Most of the storylines in my sample improve over the course of the series, including adversaries and struggling family members coming around to accept transgender characters. Examples of reparative narratives in my sample include Ben's mom (*Good Girls*) noting how happy Ben is when he switches schools. "It was like there was this whole planet called St. Anne's that [he] never knew about, where everyone is cool with [him] and they play hacky sack." Theo (*Chilling Adventures of Sabrina*) finds an accepting and loving romantic partner, even if he is a hobgoblin. When Unique (*Glee*) asks Coach Beiste if he has any regrets about his chest masculinization surgery, he responds, "Not for a second. That feeling of relief I have now, of finally being who I've always wanted to be, it's the best thing that's ever happened to me." In order to make Beiste feel not so alone in the process, Unique (via producer Ryan Murphy) arranged for a 300-member transgender choir to sing at McKinley High and share his experience.

According to Bendix (2020), there is a correlation between the scarcity of transmasculine roles and the limited number of transmasculine television producers. The inclusion of more transgender individuals in writers' rooms and transgender actors playing transgender roles means more of their stories will be told and told accurately. From my analysis of published interviews with writers and producers, it appears there is a strong desire to get portrayals right. When there are so few voices, however, it puts an undue burden on transgender writers and actors to represent. Rhys Ernst, a transgender filmmaker, found that nearly all portrayals incorporate the same kind of transgender coming out story (cited in Fallon, 2019). He added, "We're so overdue for any kind of trans content that's not terrible that there's this feeling like it needs to represent everybody all at once—and the exact way that will satisfy everybody's overdue need." Sepinwall (2019) optimistically noted that, although the number of LGBTQ characters on television is still low, shows are past the one-size-fits-all era. For example, *Transparent* did not have to represent all trans experience (Halberstam, 2018) in the same way *The L Word* no longer had to be "all things to all lesbians" (Sepinwall, 2019). "Perhaps we can agree that we will not expect one person, one film, one story to represent the vastly different, extremely complex and beautiful variety of our lives," according to filmmaker Jules Rosskam (cited in heinz, 2016).

Breakthrough transgender actors like Phelan and Fletcher add authenticity to their roles, not just through the legitimacy that their personal understandings bring to the characters, but also by offering viewers who may not know any transgender people an intimate look at the range of struggles and the variety of everyday experiences of transgender individuals. In this way, the discrimination endured by the transgender characters adds significantly to the audience's ability to empathize with various individuals. Viewers see characters as more than just their transitions or their gender identities and learn to differentiate gender expression from gender performance displayed in cross-dressing comedies.

Added to the pressure on television writers and producers to get stories right is the expectation that transgender individuals must educate others. An earlier episode of *Work in Progress* demonstrated the burden. Abby's brother-in-law asks her to explain her transgender boyfriend or, as he put it, "this new person you're dating." Abby lectures him, "It's not the job of the queer community to teach the straight cis community . . . Read a book!" (Sepinwall, 2019). Gender-diverse actors have appreciated being consulted on set; however, producers and writers may be placing an undue burden on transgender people to instruct others. Elements (2018) argued, "[W]hen the expectation is on trans people to teach others about our experiences—and not on others to educate themselves before interacting with us—we're being asked to do additional emotional labor and we're not being treated just like everyone else." Transgender actor Elliot Fletcher expressed gratitude that the writers wanted his feedback, but at the same time he thought, "Wow, is this my job? I don't know if I want this to be my job. I just want to come on set and be able to act because I love to act" (Whitney, 2017). As far as advice to writers and directors asking transgender actors questions, Fletcher added, "Please, go on the internet, contact GLAAD. There are so many things that you could do without insulting or getting way too personal with me" (Whitney, 2017). Danny M. Lavery (2021) advised *Dear Prudence* podcast listeners not to instrumentalize other people. For example, do not grab a transgender person and say, "It's your job to make me a better person. Please explain your life to me."

Appendix

Character Chart

Year 1st Appeared	*Actor Name*	*Character Name*	*Series*	*Network*
2000	Matt O'Toole	Paul	*CSI: Crime Scene Investigation*	CBS
2006	Daniela Sea	Max	*The L Word*	Showtime
2010	Jordan Todosey	Adam	*Degrassi: The Next Generation*	TeenNick
2010	Dot-Marie Jones	Sheldon	*Glee*	FOX
2014	Bex Taylor-Klaus	Lex	*House of Lies*	Showtime
2014	Tom Phelan	Cole	*The Fosters*	Freeform
2014	Ian Harvie	Dale	*Transparent*	Prime
2016	Hannah Allgood	Frankie	*Better Things*	FX
2016	Jamie Bloch	Yael	*Degrassi: Next Class*	Netflix
2016	Ian Alexander	Buck	*The OA*	Netflix
2016	Elliot Fletcher	Noah	*Faking It*	MTV
2016	Elliot Fletcher	Aaron	*The Fosters*	Freeform
2016	Zelda Williams	Drew	*Dead of Summer*	Freeform
2016	Elliot Fletcher	Trevor	*Shameless*	Showtime
2016	Asia Kate Dillion	Taylor	*Billions*	Showtime
2016	Ian Harvie	Michael	*Mistresses*	ABC
2017	Maren Heary	Dolly	*Gypsy*	Netflix
2017	Alex Blue Davis	Casey	*Grey's Anatomy*	ABC
2017	Brian Michael Smith	Toine	*Queen Sugar*	OWN
2018	Isaiah Stannard	Ben	*Good Girls*	NBC
2018	Sheridan Pierce	Syd	*One Day at a Time*	Netflix
2018	Ellie Desautels	Michael	*Rise*	NBC
2018	Lachlan Watson	Theo	*Chilling Adventures of Sabrina*	Netflix

Year 1st Appeared	*Actor Name*	*Character Name*	*Series*	*Network*
2019	J. J. Hawkins	Riley	*Red Line*	CBS
2019	Logan Rozos	Star	*David Makes Man*	OWN
2019	Theo Germaine	James	*The Politician*	Netflix
2019	Garcia	Jake	*Tales of the City*	Netflix
2019	Leo Sheng	Micah	*The L Word: Generation Q*	Showtime
2019	Bex Taylor-Klaus	Bishop	*Deputy*	FOX
2019	Daisy Eagan	Joey	*Good Trouble*	Freeform
2019	River Butcher	Lindsay	*Good Trouble*	Freeform
2019	Brian Michael Smith	Pierce	*The L Word: Generation Q*	Showtime
2020	Blue Chapman	JJ	*Council of Dads*	NBC
2020	Blu del Barrio	Adira	*Star Trek: Discovery*	Paramount +
2020	Ian Alexander	Gray	*Star Trek: Discovery*	Paramount +
2020	Theo Germaine	Chris	*Work in Progress*	Showtime
2020	Garcia	Matthew	*Party of Five (2020)*	Freeform
2020	Brian Michael Smith	Paul	*9-1-1 Lone Star*	FOX
2020	E. R. Fightmaster	Em	*Shrill*	Hulu
2021	Dua Saleh	Cal	*Sex Education*	Netflix
2021	Robyn Holdaway	Layla	*Sex Education*	Netflix
2021	J. J. Hawkins	Kevin	*Charmed*	CW
2021	Elliot Fletcher	Sam	*Y: The Last Man*	FX
2021	E. R. Fightmaster	Kai	*Grey's Anatomy*	ABC

References

Abrams, M. (2019, November 21). Is there a difference between being transgender and transsexual? *Healthline*. Retrieved from www.healthline.com/health/transgender/difference-between-transgender-and-transsexual

Abrams, M. (2020, January 27). Gender essentialism is flawed: Here's why. *Healthline*. Retrieved from www.healthline.com/health/gender-essentialism#definition

Adams, N. (2016, September 1). Men who play transgender women send a "toxic and dangerous" message. *The Hollywood Reporter*. Retrieved from www.hollywoodreporter.com/news/matt-bomer-transgender-movie-anything-guest-column-925170

Adams, N. (2020, September 2). Meet Star Trek: Discovery's Blue del Barrio. *GLAAD*. Retrieved from www.glaad.org/blog/meet-star-trek-discoverys-blu-del-barrio

Advocate. (2011a, September 29). *Op-ed: What teaches us about labels*. Retrieved from www.advocate.com/politics/commentary/2011/09/29/what-albert-nobbs-teaches-us-about-labels

Advocate. (2011b, December 28). *Op-ed: 14 reasons that made 2011 great for trans people*. Retrieved from www.advocate.com/society/transgendered/2011/12/28/14-reasons-made-2011-great-trans-people?page=0,11

Allen, S. (2017, May 5). Transgender "survivor" contestant Zeke Smith outed on national television. *Daily Beast*. Retrieved from www.thedailybeast.com/transgender-survivor-contestant-zeke-smith-outed-on-national-television

Anderson, T. (2015, December 18). Visibility matters: Transgender characters on film and television through the years. *Los Angeles Times*. Retrieved from https://timelines.latimes.com/transgender-characters-film-tv-timeline/

August, H. M. (2019, August 9). Showrunner Aaron Martin talks Netflix's another life. *TV Goodness*. Retrieved from www.tvgoodness.com/2019/08/09/showrunner-aaron-martin-talks-netflixs-another-life-exclusive/

Bandura, A. (2001). Social cognitive theory of mass communication. *Media Psychology*, *3*, 265–299.

Bastidas, J. (2019, July 3). "Good trouble" star Daisy Eagan details how the industry has improved with LGBTQ representation. *Pop Culture*. Retrieved from https://popculture.com/tv-shows/news/good-trouble-daisy-eagan-details-how-industry-improved-lgbtq-representation/

Beirne, R. (2013). The T word: Exploring transgender representation in *The L Word*. In D. Heller (Ed.), *Loving the L word: The complete series in focus* (pp. 23–36). London and New York, NY: I.B. Tauris.

Bem, S. L. (1981). Gender schema theory: A cognitive account of sex typing. *Psychological Review*, *88*, 354–364.

Bendix, T. (2020, October 9). How a new class of trans male actors are changing the face of television. *Time*. Retrieved from https://time.com/5686290/transgender-men-representation-television/

Berger, A. A. (1993). *An anatomy of humor*. New Brunswick, NJ: Transaction Publishers.

Berlyne, D. E. (1972). Humor and its kin. In J. H. Goldstein, & P. E. McGhee (Eds.), *The psychology of humor* (pp. 43–60). New York, NY: Academic.

Berman, M. (2015, April 29). Bruce Jenner *20/20* interview rises to over 20-million viewers. *TV Media Insights*. Retrieved from https://deadline.com/2015/04/bruce-jenner-interview-ratings-diane-sawyer-20-20-1201416149/

Bhattacharji, A. (2019, August 14). Why Brad Falchuk is Hollywood's best-kept secret. *Wall Street Journal*. Retrieved from https://www.wsj.com/articles/brad-falchuk-hollywoods-secret-11565699672

Billard, T. J. (2016). Writing in the margins: Mainstream news media representations of transgenderism. *International Journal of Communication*, *10*, 4193–4218.

Blair, K. L. (2019, June 16). Are trans people excluded from the world of dating? New research explores the extent to which trans people are excluded from dating. *Psychology Today*. Retrieved from www.psychologytoday.com/us/blog/inclusive-insight/201906/are-trans-people-excluded-the-world-dating

Blair, K. L., & Hoskin, R. A. (2019). Transgender exclusion from the world of dating: Patterns of acceptance and rejection of hypothetical trans dating partners as a function of sexual and gender identity. *Journal of Social and Personal*, *36*(7), 2074–2095.

Booth, E. T. (2011). Queering *Queer Eye*: The stability of gay identity confronts the liminality of trans embodiment. *Western Journal of Communication*, *75*(2), 185–204.

Booth, E. T. (2015). The provisional acknowledgement of identity claims in televised documentary. In L. G. Spencer, & J. Capuzza (Eds.), *Transgender communication: Histories, trends, and trajectories* (pp. 111–126). Lanham, MD: Lexington Books.

Bornstein, K., & Garber, M. (2008). Children's literature and the cultural discourse of cross-dressing. In V. Flanagan (Ed.), *Into the closet: Cross-dressing and the gendered body in children's literature* (pp. 1–17). New York, NY: Routledge.

Boucher, G. (2019, May 21). With record number of shows on air, super-producer Greg Berlanti brings needed representation to the small screen. *Deadline*. Retrieved from https://deadline.com/2019/05/greg-berlanti-disruptors-interview-news-1202610014/

Bowell, T. (n.d.). Feminist standpoint theory. *Internet Encyclopedia of Philosophy*. Retrieved December 14, 2021, from https://iep.utm.edu/fem-stan/

Burns, K. (2019, February 11). TV's second chance for trans representation: The right way. *Wired*. Retrieved from www.wired.com/story/tv-trans-representation/

Butler, J. (1990). *Gender trouble*. New York, NY: Routledge.

Capuzza, J. C., & Spencer, L. G. (2017). Regressing, progressing, or transgressing on the small screen? Transgender characters on U.S. scripted television series. *Communication Quarterly, 65*(2), 214–230. https://doi.org/:10.1080/01463373.2016.1221438.

Cavalcante, A. (2018). *Struggling for ordinary: Media and transgender belonging in everyday life*. New York, NY: NYU Press.

CBC. (2021, April 2). Q&A—Evie MacDonald on playing a transgender teen in new series First Day. *CBC Kids News*. Retrieved from www.cbc.ca/kidsnews/post/qa-evie-macdonald-on-playing-a-transgender-teen-in-new-series-first-day

Charles, R. (Host). (2021, March 19). Pop! Goes the queens. (Season 13 Episode 12) [TV series episode]. In S. Corfe (Executive Producer), *RuPaul's Drag Race*. World of Wonder.

Chuba, K. (2018, July 18). Ryan Murphy on "showrunning as advocacy" and the post-Me Too "age of enlightenment". *Variety*. Retrieved from https://variety.com/2018/scene/news/ryan-murphy-ronan-farrow-showrunning-as-advocacy-1202877298/

Clark, C. C. (1969). Television and social control: Some observations on the portrayals of ethnic minorities. *Television Quarterly*, 8, 18–22.

Craig, S. L., McInroy, L., McCready, L. T., & Alaggia, R. (2015). Media: A catalyst for resilience in lesbian, gay, bisexual, transgender, and queer youth. *Journal of LGBT Youth, 12*, 254–275. http://doi.org/10.1080/19361653.2015.1040193

Cuby, M. (2019, March 22). *The OA's* Ian Alexander explains why Hollywood has no excuse not to cast trans actors. *Them*. Retrieved from www.them.us/story/ian-alexander-interview

Damshenas, S. (2021). Gottmik opens up for the first time about being a trans male drag queen. *Gay Times (UK)*. Retrieved from www.gaytimes.co.uk/amplify/gottmik-opens-up-for-the-first-time-about-being-a-trans-male-drag-queen-amplify-by-gay-times/

Davidmann, S. (2010). Beyond borders. In S. Hines, & T. Sanger (Eds.), *Transgender identities: Towards a social analysis of gender diversity* (pp. 186–203). New York, NY: Routledge.

Donaghue, E. (2020, July 14). "Horrific spike" in fatal violence against transgender community. *CBS News*. Retrieved from www.cbsnews.com/news/transgender-community-fatal-violence-spike/

Douglas, S. J. (2010). *The rise of enlightened sexism: How pop culture took us from girl power to girls gone wild*. New York, NY: Henry Holt and Company.

Dry, J. (2019, June 19). How Ryan Murphy's "showrunning as advocacy" led to Janet Mock's historic Netflix deal. *Indy Wire*. Retrieved from www.indiewire.com/2019/06/ryan-murphy-pose-interview-janet-mock-lgbt-1202151338/

Edwards, M. (2010). Transconversations: New media and community. In C. Pullen & M. Cooper (Eds.), *LGBT identity and online new media* (pp. 159–172). London, UK: Routledge Press.

Ehren, A. (2015, November 8). Trans visibility: Who is it good for? *The Huffington Post*. Retrieved from www.huffpost.com/entry/trans-visibility-who-is-i_b_10310268

Ehrensaft, D. (2016, February 2). Look at him, he's Sandra Dee: What House of Lies' Roscoe can teach us about gender-nonconforming children. *Huffington Post*. Retrieved from www.huffpost.com/entry/house-of-lies-roscoe_b_1232036

Elements, K. C. (2018, June 20). *Queer Eye* is still failing trans men. *Into*. Retrieved from www.intomore.com/culture/queer-eye-is-still-failing-trans-men/

Ellis, S. K. (2020). GLAAD: Where we are on TV 2019–2020. *GLAAD Media Institute*. Retrieved from www.glaad.org/whereweareontv19

Ennis, D. (2015, September 30). What's the story behind the "transgender tragedy" on *Law & Order: SVU*? *Advocate*. Retrieved from www.advocate.com/arts-entertainment/2015/9/30/whats-story-behind-transgender-tragedy-tonights-law-order-svu

Fallon, K. (2019, August 13). Inside "Adam," the movie LGBT activists want banned, and the perils of trans storytelling in 2019. *Daily Beast*. Retrieved from www.thedailybeast.com/inside-adam-the-trans-movie-lgbt-activists-want-banned-and-the-perils-of-trans-storytelling-in-2019

Feder, S. (Director). (2020). *Disclosure* [Film]. Disclosure Films.

Fitzpatrick, K. (2016, September 30). Real "Portlandia" feminist bookstore slams the show as offensive. *Screen Crush*. Retrieved from https://screencrush.com/portlandia-feminist-bookstore-statement/

Framke, C. (2018, March 7). How RuPaul's comments on trans women led to a Drag Race revolt—and a rare apology. *Vox*. Retrieved from www.vox.com/culture/2018/3/6/17085244/rupaul-trans-women-drag-queens-interview-controversy

Freud, S. (1928). Humor. *International Journal of Psychoanalysis*, *9*, 1–6.

Friedland, W. (2018, June 5). "Good Girls" among shows with young characters exploring their gender. *Variety*. Retrieved from https://variety.com/2018/tv/awards/good-girls-billions-non-binary-characters-1202829537/

Gallagher, N. M., & Bodenhausen, G. V. (2021). Gender essentialism and the mental representation of transgender women and men: A multimethod investigation of stereotype content. *Cognition*, *217*. https://doi.org/10.1016/j.cognition.2021.104887

Gamson, J. (2001). Talking freaks: Lesbian, gay, bisexual and transgendered families on day-time talk TV. In M. Bernstein, & R. Reimann (Eds.), *Queer families, queer politics: Challenging culture and the state* (pp. 68–86). New York, NY: Columbia University Press.

Garratt, S. (2012, May 22). Chloë Sevigny interview for "*Hit & Miss*" on Sky Atlantic. *The Telegraph*. Retrieved from https://www.telegraph.co.uk/culture/tvandradio/9267261/Chloe-Sevigny-interview-for-Hit-and-Miss-on-Sky-Atlantic.html

Garrett, A. (2019, May 10). Isaiah Stannard on *Good Girls* is getting the coming-out storyline all trans kids deserve. *Distractify*. Retrieved from www.distractify.com/p/isaiah-stannard-good-girls

Generations. (n.d.). *IMDB*. Retrieved December 14, 2021, from www.imdb.com/title/tt4158624/

Gerbner, G. (1998). Cultivation analysis: An overview. *Mass Communication and Society*, *1*(3–4), 175–194.

Gerbner, G., & Gross, L. (1976). Living with television. *Journal of Communication*, *26*, 172–199.

Gersen, J. S. (2016). The transgender bathroom debate and the looming Title IX crisis. *The New Yorker*. Retrieved from www.newyorker.com/news/news-desk/public-bathroom-regulations-could-create-a-title-ix-crisis

GLAAD (2020, April 28). *GLAAD chats with the Chapman family about NBC's "Council of Dads"*. Retrieved from www.glaad.org/blog/glaad-chats-chapman-family-about-nbcs-council-dads

GLAAD (n.d.). *Victims or villains: Examining ten years of transgender images on television*. Retrieved December 14, 2021, from www.glaad.org/publications/victims-or-villains-examining-ten-years-transgender-images-television

Goldberg, L. (2018, January 18). How "Grey's Anatomy" wants to change the portrayal of trans characters on TV. *Hollywood Reporter*. Retrieved from www.hollywoodreporter.com/tv/tv-news/greys-anatomy-transgender-storyline-explained-alex-blue-davis-interview-1075535/

Goldstein, J. (1976). Theoretical notes on humor. *Journal of Communication, 26*(3), 104–112.

Gouttebroze, M. (2013). First annual studio responsibility index finds lack of substantial LGBT characters in mainstream films. *GLAAD*. Retrieved from www.glaad.org/blog/first-annual-studio-responsibility-index-finds-lack-substantial-lgbt-characters-mainstream

Grant, J. M., Mottet, L. A., & Tanis, J. (2011). Injustice at every turn: A report of the national transgender discrimination survey. *National Center for Transgender Equality and National Gay and Lesbian Task Force*. Retrieved from https://transequality.org/sites/default/files/docs/resources/NTDS_Report.pdf

Green, J. (2016). FTM: An emerging voice. In D. Denny (Ed.), *Current concepts in transgender identity* (p. 145–161). New York, NY: Routledge.

Halberstam, J. (1998). *Female masculinity*. Durham, NC: Duke University.

Halberstam, J. (2018). *Trans*: A quick and quirky account of gender variability*. Berkeley, CA: University of California Press.

Halberstam, J. J. (2005). *In a queer time and place: Transgender bodies, subcultural lives (sexual cultures)*. New York, NY: NYU Press.

Halpern, M. (2019). Feminist standpoint theory and science communication. *Journal of Science Communication, 18*(4), C02.

Hansen, C. (2021, April 9). Republican state lawmakers push wave of bills targeting transgender youth. *US News*. Retrieved from www.usnews.com/news/national-news/articles/2021-04-09/republican-state-lawmakers-push-wave-of-bills-targeting-transgender-youth

Harding, S. (2004). *The feminist standpoint theory reader*. New York, NY: Routledge.

Hassanein, R. (2018, September 12). New study reveals shocking rates of attempted suicide among trans adolescents. *Human Rights Campaign*. Retrieved from www.hrc.org/blog/new-study-reveals-shocking-rates-of-attempted-suicide-among-trans-adolescen

heinz, m. (2012). Transmen on the web: Inscribing multiple discourses. In K. Rose (Ed.), *The handbook of gender, sex, and media* (pp. 326–343). Chichester, UK: John Wiley & Sons.

heinz, m. (2016). *Entering transmasculinity: The inevitability of discourse*. Chicago, IL: University of Chicago Press.

Henderson, T. (2018, February 6). Elliot Fletcher on coming out misconceptions, trans rights, & immigration reform on *The Fosters*. *Pride*. Retrieved from www.pride.com/tv/2018/2/06/elliot-fletcher-coming-out-misconceptions-trans-rights-immigration-reform-fosters

Henry, C. (2019, October). The swash of the trans new wave. *Senses of Cinema*. Retrieved from www.sensesofcinema.com/2019/cinema-in-the-2010s/the-swash-of-the-trans-new-wave/

Hobbes, T. (1651/1909). *Leviathan*. Oxford, UK: Clarendon Press.

Holder, S. (2019, August 20). Why there's a homelessness crisis among transgender teens. *Bloomberg*. Retrieved from www.bloomberg.com/news/articles/2019-08-20/how-transgender-youth-can-escape-homelessness

Hsieh, H., & Shannon, S. (2005). Three approaches to qualitative content analysis. *Qualitative Health Research, 15*(9), 1277–1288.

Jackson, K. (2020, July 7). After backlash, Halle Berry backs out of potential role as transgender character. *Showbiz CheatSheet*. Retrieved from www.cheatsheet.com/entertainment/after-backlash-halle-berry-backs-out-of-potential-role-as-transgender-character.html/

Jones, J. M. (2021, February 24). LGBT identification rises to 5.6% in latest U.S. estimate. *Gallup*. Retrieved from https://news.gallup.com/poll/329708/lgbt-identification-rises-latest-estimate.aspx

Kaspar, B. J. (2018, July 6). Skyler Jay reveals his true feelings on *Queer Eye*'s trans makeover episode. *Them*. Retrieved from www.them.us/story/skyler-jay-reveals-his-true-feelings-on-queer-eyes-trans-makeover-episode

Keegan, C. M. (2013, June 1). Moving bodies: Sympathetic migrations in transgender narrativity. *Genders*. Retrieved from www.colorado.edu/gendersarchive 1998-2013/2013/06/01/moving-bodies-sympathetic-migrations-transgender-narrativity

Kellner, D. (1995). Cultural studies, multiculturalism and media culture. In G. Dines, & J. Humez (Eds.), *Gender, race and class in media* (pp. 5–17). Thousand Oaks, CA: Sage.

Kelso, T. (2015). Still trapped in the U.S. media's closet: Representations of gender-variant, pre-adolescent children. *Journal of Homosexuality, 62*(8), 1058–1097.

Kerry, S. (2009). "There's genderqueers on the starboard bow": The pregnant male in *Star Trek*. *Journal of Popular Culture, 42*(4), 699–714.

King, S. (2019, October 25). Hilary Swank reflects on *Boys Don't Cry*: It's such an important story for people to know. *The Hollywood Reporter*. Retrieved from www.hollywoodreporter.com/movies/movie-news/hilary-swank-reflects-boys-dont-cry-an-important-story-people-know-1249896/

Kornhaber, S. (2016). *Modern Family* tip-toes around its first transgender character. *The Atlantic*. Retrieved from www.theatlantic.com/entertainment/archive/2016/09/modern-family-a-stereotypical-day-transgender-child-actor-jackson-millarker/502196/

Lambert, M. (2016). Exclusive: Transgender actor Ian Harvie talks new role on "Mistresses". *Out Magazine*. Retrieved from www.out.com/out-exclusives/2016/6/19/exclusive-transgender-actor-ian-harvie-talks-new-role-mistresses

Lang, N. (2019a, May 3). How trans actors are rewriting the rules of TV casting. *New York Times*.

Lang, N. (2019b, September 12). How starring in a Netflix show helped this nonbinary actor thrive. *Out*. Retrieved from www.out.com/television/2019/9/12/how-starring-netflix-show-helped-nonbinary-actor-thrive

Lasky, M. (2021, January 14). GLAAD'S where we are on TV 2020–2021 report: Despite tumultuous year in television LGBTQ representation holds steady. *GLAAD*. Retrieved from https://www.glaad.org/releases/glaads-where-we-are-tv-2020-2021-report-despite-tumultuous-year-television-lgbtq

Lavery, D. M. (Host). (2021, February 21). Unsafe word [Audio podcast episode]. In *Dear Prudence*. Slate. Retrieved from https://slate.com/podcasts/dear-prudence/2021/02/girlfriend-doesnt-respect-safe-word-dear-prudence-advice

Leighton-Dure, S. (2019, July 31). Australian actor JayR Tinaco's role in "Another Life" helped them come out as non-binary. *SBS Australia*. Retrieved from www.sbs.com.au/topics/pride/agenda/article/2019/07/30/australian-actor-jayr-tinacos-role-another-life-helped-them-come-out-non-binary

Love, A. (2020, September 9). Allies, accomplices, and saviors: Knowing the difference to maximize impact. *Berrett-Koehler Publishers*. Retrieved from https://ideas.bkconnection.com/allies-accomplices-saviors-knowing-the-difference-to-maximize-impact

Mackie, D. (2016, May 13). Meet Elliot Fletcher, TV's first trans teen heartthrob. *Frontiers Media*. Retrieved from www.frontiersmedia.com/gay-entertainment/2016/05/13/75185/

Malcon, M. (2020, May 1). Teary-eyed Pamela Adlon gets champagne surprise from her kids for *Better Things* season finale. *Variety*. Retrieved from https://variety.com/2020/film/news/pamela-adlon-better-things-season-4-finale-gender-fluidity-1234595376/

Marzano-Lesnevich, A. (2021, June 13). The healing power of queer coming-of-age stories. *New York Times*. Retrieved from www.nytimes.com/2021/06/13/opinion/trans-queer-ya-books-film-pride.html

Master Class (2021, September 29). The differences between writing for TV versus writing for film. *Master Class*. Retrieved from www.masterclass.com/articles/the-differences-between-writing-for-tv-versus-writing-for-film#5-differences-between-television-writing-and-film-writing

McCabe, A. (2019, October 21). 20 years later, *Boys Don't Cry* still inspires admiration and debate. *NPR All Things Considered*. Retrieved from www.npr.org/2019/10/21/771451650/20-years-later-boys-don-t-cry-still-inspires-admiration-and-debate

McDonald, J. (2015, April 22). Rhys Ernst on the underrepresentation of trans-masculinity. *Out*. Retrieved from www.out.com/art-books/2015/4/22/rhys-ernst-underrepresentation-transmasculinity

McInroy, L. B., & Craig, S. L. (2015). Transgender representation in offline and online media: LGBTQ youth perspectives. *Journal of Human Behavior in the Social Environment*, *25*(6), 606–617.

McInroy, L. B., & Craig, S. L. (2017). Perspectives of LGBTQ emerging adults on the depiction and impact of LGBTQ media representation. *Journal of Youth Studies*, *20*(1), 32–46.

Merriam-Webster's Dictionary. (2021a). *Drama*. Retrieved December 14, 2021, from www.merriam-webster.com/dictionary/drama

Merriam-Webster's Dictionary. (2021b). *Masculine*. Retrieved December 14, 2021, from www.merriam-webster.com/dictionary/masculine

Metz, N. (2019, December 4). After quitting Hollywood Chicago native and co-creator of *The Matrix* Lilly Wachowski is back and this time she's shifted to comedy with Showtime's *Work in Progress*. *Chicago Tribune*. Retrieved from www.chicagotribune.com/entertainment/tv/ct-mov-work-in-progress-showtime-comedy-1206-20191204-4iuai4h63rf5pjemhtndqtnruy-story.html

Mey (2015, January 17). A tale of two trans characters: Glee's trans representation problem. *Autostraddle*. Retrieved from www.autostraddle.com/a-tale-of-two-trans-characters-glees-trans-representation-problem-273108/

Middlebrook, D. (1998). *Suits me: The double life of Billy Tipton*. Boston, MA: Houghton Mifflin.

Miller, D. (Director). (2016, September 23). Whoopie Goldberg. (Season 9, episode 5) [TV series episode]. In R. Dauber (Executive Producer), *The Wendy Williams show*. CBS Media Ventures.

Miller, L. J. (2015). Becoming one of the girls/guys: Distancing transgender representations in popular film comedies. In J. C. Capuzza, & L. G. Spencer (Eds.), *Transgender communication studies: Histories, trends, and trajectories* (pp. 127–142). Lanham, MD: Lexington Books.

Minkin, R., & Brown, A. (2021, July 27). Rising shares of U.S. adults know someone who is transgender or goes by gender-neutral pronouns. *Pew Research*. Retrieved from www.pewresearch.org/fact-tank/2021/07/27/rising-shares-of-u-s-adults-know-someone-who-is-transgender-or-goes-by-gender-neutral-pronouns/

Mitovich, M. W. (2021, January 14). GLAAD: TV's LGBTQ representation dipped amid pandemic, because too few shows do too much of the work. *TV Line*. Retrieved from https://tvline.com/2021/01/14/glaad-report-tv-lgbtq-representation-down-during-pandemic/

Mocarski, R., Butler, S., Emmons, B., & Smallwood, R. (2013). A different kind of man: Mediated transgendered subjectivity, Chaz Bono on *Dancing with the Stars*. *Journal of Communication Inquiry*, *37*(3), 249–264.

Molloy, P. M. (2014, March 3). Tom Phelan breaks ground as trans actor playing trans teen on *The Fosters*. *Pride*. Retrieved from www.pride.com/television/2014/03/03/exclusive-tom-phelan-breaks-ground-trans-actor-playing-trans-teen-osters

Montes, G. (2012, December 11). Shonda Rhimes defends LGBT visibility on TV. *GLAAD*. Retrieved from https://www.glaad.org/blog/shonda-rhimes-defends-lgbt-visibility-tv

Morgan, S. E., Harrison, T. R., Chewning, L., Davis, L., & Dicorcia, M. (2007). Entertainment (mis) education: The framing of organ donation in entertainment television. *Health Communication*, *22*(2), 143–151.

Morreall, J. (1983). *Taking laughter seriously*. Albany, NY: SUNY Press.

Moscovici, S. (1973). Foreword. In C. Herzlich (Ed.), *Health and illness: A social psychological analysis* (pp. ix–xiv). New York, NY: Academic Press.

Murchison, G. (2017, March 31). New HRC poll: Improving favorability toward transgender people. *Human Rights Campaign*. Retrieved from www.hrc.org/blog/new-hrc-poll-improving-favorability-toward-transgender-people

Nichols, L. (2018, July 5). *Pose* co-creator on the show's groundbreaking authenticity. *Philadelphia Gay News*.

Noble, B. J. (2004). *Masculinities without men*. Vancouver, BC: UBC Press.

Oliver, D. (2020, November 24). Hollywood's casting dilemma: Should straight, cisgender actors play LGBTQ characters? *USA Today*. Retrieved from www.usatoday.com/story/entertainment/celebrities/2020/11/24/should-straight-cisgender-actors-play-lgbtq-characters-in-hollywood/6327858002/

Oppliger, P. A. (2008). *Girls gone skank: Sexual representations of girls in American culture*. Jefferson, NC: McFarland Publishing.

Oppliger, P. A., & Medeiros, M. (2017). Free to be he: Portrayals of transgendered characters in Freeform's *The Fosters*. *A paper presented at the Eastern Communication Association Conference*, Boston, MA.

Paley, A. (2020). National survey on LGBTQ youth mental health 2020. *The Trevor Project*. Retrieved from www.thetrevorproject.org/survey-2020/

Palmer, L. (2015). *The Fosters* star on the rise of transgender television: "It's not going to do a lot". *The Hollywood Reporter*. Retrieved from www.hollywoodreporter.com/live-feed/fosters-transgender-tom-phelan-interview-808424

Parkinson, H. J. (2015, June 2). Caitlyn Jenner smashes Twitter world record, reaching a million followers. *The Guardian*. Retrieved from www.theguardian.com/technology/2015/jun/02/caitlyn-jenner-twitter-record-million-followers-vanity-fair

Phillips, J. (2006). *Transgender on the screen*. Basingstoke, UK: Palgrave MacMillan.

Poole, Ralph J. (2017). Towards a queer futurity: New trans television. *European Journal of American Studies*, *12*(2), 1–23.

Ramos, D. R. (2021, January 4). RuPaul's Drag Race season 13 premiere slays as most-watched episode in franchise's history. *Deadline*. Retrieved from https://deadline.com/2021/01/rupauls-drag-race-season-13-premiere-vh1-ratings-most-watched-episode-1234664587/

Rapaport, L. (2019, May 6). Trans teens face higher sexual assault risk when schools restrict bathrooms. *Reuters*. Retrieved from www.reuters.com/article/us-health-youth-transgender/trans-teens-face-higher-sexual-assault-risk-when-schools-restrict-bathrooms-idUSKCN1SC1LR

Real, E. (2018, June 1). Ryan Murphy says *Pose* could have never happened without trans talent. *The Hollywood Reporter*. Retrieved from www.hollywoodreporter.com/live-feed/ryan-murphy-pose-hiring-transgender-talent-1116572

Reed, J. (2009). Reading gender politics on *The L Word*: The Moira/Max transitions. *Journal of Popular Film & Television*, *37*(4), 169–178.

Riggs, D. W. (2014). What makes a man? Thomas Beatie, embodiment, and "mundane transphobia". *Feminism & Psychology*, *24*(2), 157–171.

Rigney, M. (2003). Brandon goes to Hollywood: *Boys Don't Cry* and the transgender body in film. *Film Criticism*, *28*(2), 4–23.

Ringo, P. (2002). Media roles in female-to-male transsexual and transgender identity formation. *International Journal of Transgenderism*, *6*(3), 97–103.

Rojas, M. (2017, September 29). *3 Generations* review: Not the trans youth film we were hoping for. *Cinemacy*. Retrieved from https://cinemacy.com/3-generations-is-not-the-trans-youth-film-we-were-hoping-for/

Roscoe, W. (1996). Priests of the goddess: Gender transgression in ancient religion. *History of Religions*, *35*(3), 195–230.

Sandercock, T. (2015). Transing the small screen: Loving and hating transgender youth in Glee and Degrassi. *Journal of Gender Studies*, *24*(4), 436–452.

Schenkel, H. (2015). Stuck in time: intersex and transgender representation in Predestination. *Screen Education, 79*, 54–63.

Schmider, A. (2021, July 15). In *No Ordinary Man* trans men reflect on the life of jazz musician Billy Tipton, reclaiming his place in trans history. *GLAAD*. Retrieved from www.glaad.org/blog/no-ordinary-man-trans-men-reflect-life-jazz-musician-billy-tipton-reclaiming-his-place-trans

Schmidt, S. (2020, August 17). Federal judge blocks Trump administration from ending transgender health-care protections. *Washington Post*. Retrieved from www.washingtonpost.com/dc-md-va/2020/08/17/federal-judge-blocks-trump-administration-ending-transgender-healthcare-protections/

Schneider, M. (2019, August 19). Listen: Laverne Cox on *Sex and the City's* troubling transphobia and why it's still her favorite show. *Variety*. Retrieved from https://variety.com/2019/tv/news/laverne-cox-sex-and-the-city-orange-is-the-new-black-my-favorite-episode-1203306932/

Schultz, H. (2016, October 27). A conversation with Tom Phelan. *Stage & Candor*. Retrieved from https://stageandcandor.com/conversations/tom-phelan/#.Ybi689DMJaQ

Sebastian, M. (2015, December 16). Here are the 10 most popular people of the year according to Google. *Cosmopolitan*. Retrieved from www.cosmopolitan.in/celebrity/news/g454/here-are-10-most-popular-people-year-according-google

Seid, D. M. (2014). Reveal. *Transgender Studies Quarterly*, *1*(1–2), 176–177.

Sepinwall, A. (2019, December 6). *Work in Progress* review: The dark and delightful times of a "fat, queer dyke". *Rolling Stone*. Retrieved from www.rollingstone.com/tv/tv-reviews/work-in-progress-showtime-review-920903/

Serano, J. (2007). *Whipping girl: A transsexual woman on the scapegoating of femininity*. Emeryville, CA: Seal Press.

Serano, J. (2013). Skirt chasers: Why the media depicts the trans revolution in lipstick and heels. In S. Stryker, & A. Z. Aizura (Eds.), *The transgender studies reader 2* (pp. 226–233). New York, NY: Routledge.

Serano, J. (2016, May 3). Expanding trans media representation: Why transgender actors should be cast in cisgender roles. *Gender 2.0*. Retrieved from https://medium.com/gender-2-0/expanding-trans-media-representation-why-transgender-actors-should-be-cast-in-cisgender-roles-f880cb7bb36e#.i0recy68w

Shameless. (n.d.). *IMDB*. Retrieved from www.imdb.com/title/tt1586680/

Shelley, C. (2008). *Transpeople: Repudiation, trauma, healing*. Toronto, CA: University of Toronto Press.

Siebler, K. (2010). Transqueer representations and how we educate. *Journal of LGBT Youth*, *7*(4), 320–345.

Siebler, K. (2012). Transgender transitions: Sex/gender binaries in the digital age. *Journal of Gay & Lesbian Mental Health*, *16*(1), 74–99.

Singhal, A., & Rogers, E. M. (2003). The status of entertainment-education worldwide. In A. Singhal, M. J. Cody, E. M. Rogers, & M. Sabido (Eds.), *Entertainment-education and social change: History, research, and practice* (pp. 3–20). New York, NY: Routledge.

Soloway, J. (2018). *She wants it: Desire, power, and toppling the patriarchy*. New York, NY: Crown Archetype.

Stedman, (2018, July 13). Scarlett Johansson exits trans film "Rub and Tug" amid backlash. *Variety*. Retrieved from https://variety.com/2018/film/news/scarlett-johansson-exit-rub-and-tug-trans-backlash-1202872981/

Steinbock, E. (2017). Towards trans cinema. In K. L. Hole, D. Jeleca, E. A. Kaplan, & P. Petro (Eds.), *The Routledge companion to cinema & gender* (p. 396). Milton Park, Abingdon, Oxon: Routledge.

Steinbock, E. (2019). *Shimmering images: Trans cinema, embodiment, and the aesthetics of change*. Durham, NC: Duke University Press.

Steinmetz, K. (2014, May 29). The transgender tipping point. *Time*. Retrieved from https://time.com/135480/transgender-tipping-point/.

Stryker, S. (2008). *Transgender history*. Berkeley, CA: Seal Press.

Stryker, S. (2017). *Transgender history* (2nd ed.). Berkeley, CA: Seal Press.

Stryker, S, & Currah, P. (2014). Introduction. *TSQ: Transgender Studies Quarterly*, *1*(1–2), 1–18.

Suleman, N. (2019, June 25). Young Americans are increasingly "uncomfortable" with LGBTQ community, GLAAD study shows. *Time*. Retrieved from https://time.com/5613276/glaad-acceptance-index-lgbtq-survey/

Thomson, M. (2017, February 2). Drag: The device that makes Portlandia what it is. *Spider Web Show Performance*. Retrieved from https://spiderwebshow.ca/drag-the-device-that-makes-portlandia-what-it-is/

Transgender identity terms and labels. (n.d.). *Planned parenthood*. Retrieved December 14, 2021, from www.plannedparenthood.org/learn/gender-identity/transgender

Tsai, W. H. S. (2010). Assimilating the queers: Representations of lesbians, gay men, bisexual, and transgender people in mainstream advertising. *Advertising & Society Review*, *11*(1).

Turban, J. (2020, November). What is gender dysphoria? *American Psychiatric Association*. Retrieved from www.psychiatry.org/patients-families/gender-dysphoria/what-is-gender-dysphoria

Turchiano, D. (2018, September 18). 'Central Park' writer launches 'Show Us Your Room' social media initiative. *Variety*. Retrieved from https://variety.com/2018/tv/features/show-us-your-room-social-media-initiative-1202939127/

Ulaby, N. (2014, April 23). On television, more transgender characters come into focus. *NPR Pop Culture Happy Hour*. Retrieved from www.npr.org/transcripts/306166533

Valenza, R. (2014, Jan 10). Bradley Bredeweg, executive producer, discusses ABC Family's *The Fosters*. *The Huffington Post*. Retrieved from www.huffingtonpost.com/2014/01/10/bradley-bredeweg-the-fosters_n_4569014.html

Vary, A. B. (2020, November 6). Inside the groundbreaking *Star Trek: Discovery* episode with trans and non-binary characters. *Variety*. Retrieved from https://variety.com/2020/tv/news/star-trek-discovery-trans-non-binary-blu-del-barrio-ian-alexander-1234824183/

Veatch, T. C. (1998). A theory of humor. *Humor*, *11*(2), 161–215.

Villarreal, D. (2020, March 26). These 10 trans male TV characters represent the best (and worst) of queer TV tropes. *Hornet*. Retrieved from https://hornet.com/stories/10-trans-male-tv-characters-tropes/

Visage, M. (2021, April 13). Gottmik. [Video] *Whatcha packing*. Retrieved from www.youtube.com/watch?v=L2Y8UzxluVE

Wagner, W., Universitit, J. K., Duveen, G., & Gene, D. (1999). Theory and method of social representations. *Asian Journal of Social Psychology*, *2*, 95–125.

Walters, S. D. (2014). *Tolerance trap: How god, genes, and good intentions are sabotaging gay equality*. New York, NY: NYU Press.

Westcott, L. (2104, May 29). Laverne Cox is the first transgender person on the cover of time. *The Atlantic*. Retrieved from www.theatlantic.com/culture/archive/2014/05/laverne-cox-is-the-first-transgender-person-on-the-cover-of-time/371798/

Whitney, E. O. (2017, June 23). Don't ask shameless star Elliot Fletcher about his backstory. *ScreenCrush*. Retrieved from https://screencrush.com/elliot-fletcher-interview-our-hollywood/

Whittle, S. (2010, June 2). A brief history of transgender issues. *The Guardian*. Retrieved from www.theguardian.com/lifeandstyle/2010/jun/02/brief-history-transgender-issues\

Williams, E. R. (2018). *The screenwriter's taxonomy: A roadmap to collaborative storytelling*. New York, NY: Routledge.

Wong, C. M. (2018, January 22). Laverne Cox makes history as Cosmopolitan's first transgender cover girl. *Huffington Post*. Retrieved from www.huffpost.com/entry/laverne-cox-cosmopolitan-magazine_n_5a660054e4b0e5630071cc41

Xtra (2010, August 9). Degrassi's first trans character, Adam: Interview with actress Jordan Todosey [Video]. *Xtra*. Retrieved from www.youtube.com/watch?v=bSSdUv_R0xI

Zuckerman, E. (2015, August 17). Why *about Ray*'s director cast Elle Fanning as a trans teen. *Refinery29*. Retrieved from www.refinery29.com/en-us/2015/08/92441/about-ray-elle-fanning-poster

Index

3 Generations 6, 15–16
9-1-1 Lone Star 28, 35–36, 54, 58, 72, 87

Ace Ventura 30
Adams, Nick 16, 19, 20, 22, 52
Albert Nobbs 4, 17
Alexander, Ian 16, 19, 21, 27
Ally McBeal 25, 30, 31
Angel, Buck 39
Ashley, Laith 32, 41, 90

Banks, Tyra 38, 39
Bans, Jenna 16, 20
Berlanti, Greg 13, 14
Better Things 34, 50, 61, 88
Billions 18, 35, 36, 56–57, 69–70, 76, 83, 87
binding(s) 6, 28, 63, 66, 76, 92
Bono, Chaz 2, 10, 21, 41, 42, 57
Boys Don't Cry i, 5–6, 17, 18, 55, 79
Bredeweg, Bradley 15

Canals, Steven 14, 19
Cassata, Ryan 20, 22, 38, 39
casting 8, 12, 16, 17–20
Charmed 28, 75–76
Chilling Adventures of Sabrina 14, 27, 28, 43, 48, 53, 55, 57, 64, 68, 73, 75, 77, 84, 88–89, 94
cinema studies 2–3, 7
Cold Case 25
comedies 29–37
Council of Dads 15, 28, 33, 43, 60, 84–85, 87, 89

Couric, Katie 44
Cox, Laverne 2, 31, 44
CSI: Crime Scene Investigation 9, 24, 25, 45, 60
cultivation theory 7

Dallas Buyers Club 5, 17, 19, 53
Dancing with the Stars 2, 21, 41
David Makes Man 28, 54, 75
Davis, Alex Blue 15, 16, 21, 26
deadname/deadnames/deadnaming 48–49, 64, 65, 72, 77, 85
Dead of Summer 28, 64, 75, 77–78, 81, 86
Degrassi: Next Class 43–44, 49, 51–52, 55–56, 57, 62, 66, 73, 82, 88
Degrassi: The Next Generation 16, 28–29, 36, 48, 52, 53–54, 55, 56, 57, 59, 61, 63, 65–66, 68, 71, 75, 76–77, 79–80, 85, 86, 87, 88, 89–90
Deputy 25, 62, 64, 72, 82–83
Desperate Living 5
Donahue, Phil 38
dramas 24–29; crime dramas 24–25; hospital/medical/rescue dramas 25–26; speculative fiction 26–27

edu-tainment 42–44
Ernst, Rhys 13, 18, 94

Faking It 16, 28, 34, 64–65, 72, 81, 85
Falchuk, Brad 14
Fletcher, Elliot 10, 15, 19, 27, 80, 93, 94, 95

Fosters, The 15, 16, 20, 21, 28, 36–37, 42, 43, 47, 53, 54, 59, 63, 67–69, 73–74, 75, 80, 83, 85, 86, 92, 93

gender schema theory 8
Glee 14, 28, 34, 48, 49, 50–51, 54, 55, 58, 60, 61, 66–67, 78–79, 94
Glen or Glenda 4–5
Goldberg, Whoopie 93
Golden Girls 32, 33
Good Doctor, The 26
Good Girls 16, 19–20, 28, 34, 48, 55, 64, 75, 84, 94
Good Trouble 10, 15, 18, 27, 35, 62, 82
Gottmik 21, 42, 48–49, 50
Grassi, Michael 16, 18, 43
Grey's Anatomy 14–15, 16, 26, 27, 47, 64, 69
Gypsy 50, 55, 61, 67, 84, 87

Harvie, Ian 12, 16, 37, 49, 53, 59
HB2 "bathroom bill" vii
House of Lies 34, 50, 52, 57–58, 61–62

incongruity humor 29, 32–33, 36
Itty Bitty Titty Committee 5

J, Our Lady 14, 19
Jenner, Caitlyn 2
Jorgensen, Christine 2
Just One of the Guys 4

L.A. Doctors 26
Larry King Live 20, 38
Lavery, Danny M. 95
Law & Order: Special Victims Unit 24, 25, 31, 44
L Word, The 10, 19, 28, 48, 53, 54, 56, 58, 59, 60–61, 65, 69, 81, 85, 86–87, 92, 94
L Word: Generation Q, The 36, 59, 72–73, 81, 83, 86

McDonald, Evie 20–21
McEnany, Abby 15
Mistresses 16, 37, 57, 58–59, 78, 81, 89
Mock, Janet 14
Mrs. Doubtfire 17, 29
Murphy, Ryan 13–14, 26, 94

New Amsterdam 26, 44
Nip/Tuck 13, 264

OA, The 27
One Day at a Time 33, 34, 49–50, 51

Page, Elliot 2
Paige, Peter 15
Party of Five (2020) 69, 81
passing 56
Perry, Ellis David 22
Phelan, Tom 15, 21, 53, 93, 94
Phelan, Tony 15
Pinsky, Dr. Drew 38
Politician, The 27, 34
Portlandia 33
Pose 7, 9, 13, 14, 18, 19, 32
Povich, Maury 38
Preciado, Emmett 10, 21, 26

Queen Sugar 28
Queer Eye 21, 39–40, 53, 54–55, 57, 66, 69

Raphael, Sally Jesse 39
Rater, Joan 15
Ray, Carter 22
reality television 37–42; competitive shows 41–42; docu-shows 39–41; talk shows 37–39, 44
Red Line 14, 49
relief humor 29, 31–32
reparative narratives 93
Rhimes, Shonda 13, 14
Richards, Renee 2
Rise 16, 28, 48, 57, 68, 71–72, 75, 79, 84, 88
Rivera, Geraldo 38
RuPaul's Drag Race 21, 42, 48–49, 50

satire 33–34
Schofield, Scott Turner 21
Sense8 7, 19, 26–27
Sex and the City 31, 32
Sex Education 28, 34, 43, 51, 56, 66, 74, 82, 88
Shakespeare in Love 4, 17
Shameless 28, 34, 35, 42–43, 47, 52, 53, 56, 65, 69, 81, 83
She's the Man 4

Smith, Brian Michael 21, 54
Smith, Zeke 22, 41
social affirmation 46–47
social learning theory 8, 90
social representation theory 7, 10
Soloway, Joey 13
Some Like it Hot 3, 17
South Park 33–34
Springer, Jerry 37–38, 44
standpoint theory 12–13
Star Trek: Discovery 16–17, 27, 63–64
Stern, Howard 39
Strut 39, 41, 44, 90, 93
Suite Life on Deck, The 29
superiority humor 29, 30–31
Survivor 41–42, 44

Tales of the City 36, 51, 54, 58, 81, 86
talk shows *see* reality television
testosterone 19, 26, 27, 37, 39, 53–54, 55, 60, 66, 81, 85, 86, 92
This is Us 36
Tinaco, JayR 20, 21
Tipton, Billy 2, 21–22
Tootsie 17, 29
Transparent 9, 13, 18, 19, 34, 37, 53, 58, 67, 83, 94
transplaining 73, 74
Trump administration vii
Two and a Half Men 31–32, 59

Ugly Betty 31

Vernoff, Krista 16, 47, 64
Victor/Victoria 4, 17
Vilson, Marquise 21

Wachowski, Lilly 15, 26
Waithe, Lena 13, 14
Winfrey, Oprah 37, 38, 76
Work in Progress 15, 28, 34, 35, 48, 67, 83, 95
wrong body 47, 59, 61, 92

Y: The Last Man 27, 63
Yentl 4, 17

Zoey 101 29

For Product Safety Concerns and Information please contact our EU representative GPSR@taylorandfrancis.com
Taylor & Francis Verlag GmbH, Kaufingerstraße 24, 80331 München, Germany

www.ingramcontent.com/pod-product-compliance
Lightning Source LLC
LaVergne TN
LVHW010934110826
845149LV00013B/2587

* 9 7 8 1 0 3 2 0 6 8 9 9 2 *